Making Meals With Mary

Easy to prepare recipes for healthy living. Bible based scientifically sound data with explanations of phytochemicals, enzymes, and antioxidants.

by Mary Hughen

CJH Enterprises

Library of Congress Cataloging-in Publication Data 98-073871

ISBN 1-890683-02-7

Published in 1998 in the year of its copyright.

HUGHEN, Mary, Author 1942 -

    Making Meals With Mary - Easy to prepare, tasty and healthful recipes using unprocessed natural foods and flavorings. Bible based, scientifically sound nutritional data explaining phytochemicals, enzymes, and antioxidants. Also includes data as to why certain foods are harmful to the body.

Edited by the staff of CJH ENTERPRISES

Cover by Mark Glodfelter

Bulk sales for fund raising activities are available at discount prices.
Contact Mary Hughen
The Nutrition Mission
1825 Morgan Cemetery Road
Molino, FL 32577
Telephone (850) 587-5680

Printed by
PACE PRINTERS
Pensacola, Florida

Published by
CJH ENTERPRISES
6064 Mayberry Lane
Milton, Florida 32570-8875
Telephone (850) 626-2700, Fax (850) 626-7040

Printed in the United States of America

Dedication

This book is dedicated to Amy Pennay, a very good friend with whom I share my home including my kitchen. Amy has faithfully and frequently implored, "Mary, you *have* to finish your cookbook before I get married and move away. I *must* have a copy of it."

Well, here it is Amy - and thank you for the daily encouragement you gave me.

TABLE OF CONTENTS

The purpose of this book is to provide healthful tasty recipes made from natural foods. No statement or any part of this book is intended for diagnosing or prescribing. One should consult a health practitioner before deciding on any course of treatment for a condition.

Foreword

My people are destroyed for lack of knowledge. Hosea 4:8.

The above Bible verse speaks directly to me. My husband and I heard about the benefits of natural unprocessed foods in 1978. We briefly entertained thoughts of eating whole grains and using honey instead of sugar.

Then we reasoned that there was no need for us to make such a drastic change in our diet. After all, we were healthy. Not fully comprehending the concept of good health, we believed that such a diet could make sick people well. It never occurred to us that a natural diet should be followed to help healthy people maintain their good health.

Several years later, adversity struck our home. My husband had a brain tumor which the doctors said must be surgically removed. We consented. The surgery left him totally disabled. He spent nineteen days in a comatose sleep. After ten weeks in the hospital and six additional surgeries, he came home in a bedridden, lethargic condition.

We began a program of metabolic therapy and made drastic changes in our diet. His condition begin to improve. Then I consented to an advanced kind of radiation known as "fractionated stereotactic treatment," which was supposed to destroy the residual of the tumor. In doing so, it destroyed a vital portion of his brain and led to his untimely death.

The day of his death, I prayed, "Dear Lord, please don't let my husband's death have been in vain. Give me the knowledge and the strength to help others avoid the pitfalls that we stepped into."

One morning shortly thereafter, as I was reading my Bible, my eyes fell upon III John 2. Although I had read the verse many times, I had never seen it the way I saw it that morning. *Beloved, I wish above all things that thou mayest prosper and be in health, even as thy soul prospereth.* As I meditated on the message of that verse and prayed, I felt a clear calling from God to study and promote nutrition. I knew beyond any doubt that nutrition was my mission.

Several months later, I enrolled in Clayton College of Natural Health, Birmingham, Alabama, where I received my B.S. degree in Natural Health.

Please do not make the mistake that we made. If you are enjoying good health today, look at these recipes as a means of continuing good health. If you are experiencing health problems, consider these recipes as a way to nourish your body and boost your immune system.

Many of these recipes originated from my old unhealthful ones. By changing some of the ingredients, I made them into healthful dishes. You will find that you can do the same with some of your "old favorites." If some of the ingredients are unfamiliar to you, consult the glossary. As you buy groceries each week, replace your harmful food items with more nutritional foods. Do this consistently - one step at the time - and you will experience the benefits of good health! As an added bonus, your tastes and food cravings will change!

I challenge you to eat these healthful foods for six months. When you crave a candy bar, eat a piece of fruit. When you crave an unhealthful pizza, make a healthful one. When you feel that you must have a soft drink, drink water. It's called will power. Will power pays dividends of good health, and good health begins in the kitchen!

Mary Hughen

Introduction

I was diagnosed as having lupus in 1984. At that time, the doctors determined that I probably had the condition since childhood. They treated me with prednisone, and began giving me chemotherapy in August 1991. According to them, I did not have long to live. That would have been true had I continued the treatments.

In August, 1994, my friend, Mary Hughen, expressed her concerns about the adverse effects of my treatments. When she told me there was an alternative, I thought she was crazy. Had the doctors not told me that I would die if I stopped the treatments?

One evening in July 1995, I told Mary that I had to go for my next chemo treatment the following day. She answered, "No, you don't *have* to."

Again, I thought my friend was crazy. "Yes I do *have* to," I replied, as I turned and walked away. I really thought she didn't understand.

That treatment made me sicker than I had ever been. I honestly thought I would die. There was a distinctive rotten smell about me. It was too awful to put into words. Mary's words, "No, you don't *have* to," echoed through my mind again and again. While I was deathly ill, God gave me perfect peace about discontinuing my chemo.

At this point, I will tell you about my children. My nine-year-old son was taking ritalin for his attention deficit disorder. My seven-year-old daughter, who also had lupus, was taking pain medications every day and was experiencing a rapid weight loss. Our doctor wanted to treat her with prednisone, but I adamantly refused the treatment. "It will blow her up like a balloon. You see what it has done to me," I told the doctor.

One day in early September 1995, I called Mary and asked her about the alternative. I listened to her advice and acted upon it. Since then, my way of thinking and eating has totally changed. Because of Mary's diligence and because of my children begging me to stay out of the hospital, I am on the road to recovery today.

Within a few short months after our drastic change in diet, my son was able to discontinue his ritalin. His hyperactivity is controlled by diet. To the doctor's amazement, my daughter's lupus went into remission and has been totally inactive the past two years. She is the picture of health. My own immune system is healing my body. My blood work is normal, and my energy level is better than it has ever been.

If you have an illness of any kind, I strongly recommend that you choose proper diet and nutrition, thus allowing your immune system to heal your body. Begin by using Mary's recipes. If you are already healthy, discontinue those fast foods and processed foods now. Don't wait until your marvelous body that God created is loaded with toxins and filled with disease. Nourish your body with whole foods which will boost your immune system and *keep* you healthy!

Sheila Ann Menard
Pensacola, FL

Chapter 1

YOUR KITCHEN

Why Spend Time In The Kitchen?

Your kitchen can be a delightful place, yet most people do not see it as such. Why should you prepare your own meals when fast food restaurants are plentiful? Who has time to make a lunch to eat at work? Wouldn't it make more sense to walk across the street or drive three or four blocks from the office in order to get a warm meal? Wouldn't it save time to stop on the way home and pick up a box of fried chicken or a few hamburgers? Why not visit the deli section of your favorite grocery store and purchase some lunch meats and a loaf of bread? Or perhaps you are in the mood for frozen dinners this evening. Doesn't a frozen dinner of meat and vegetables provide a balanced meal?

America has become a land of fast pace and fast foods. If you are a victim of this fast society, your health as well as the health of your family is at stake. Have you considered that the time you are saving away from the kitchen might be spent in the doctor's office or in a hospital? If you could get a vision of what those quick and easy foods are doing to your body and to the bodies of those whom you love, you would most likely work some time into your busy schedule to prepare nutritional meals for yourself and for your family.

After World War II, many American women began working in factories and making quick meals for their families. Grocery store owners saw a way to make money. They stocked their shelves with canned foods which are extremely high in sodium and low in potassium, not to mention the harmful preservatives and the aluminum cans. Half a century later, doctors' offices and hospitals are filled with patients who are taking chemical drugs and undergoing surgery for their ailments because they have failed to nourish their body cells with a life giving diet.

Phytochemicals

What is the processed food diet missing? Among other things, it is missing phytochemicals. *Phyto* is derived from the Greek word *phyton,* meaning *plant.* Phytochemicals may be defined as *plant chemicals.* Because God planned and created the universe in a perfect balance, plants contain the chemicals required for the body to produce the vitamins and minerals it needs for its many functions.

Full benefit is achieved when your produce is allowed to ripen on the vine, bush, or tree and harvested when first ripe. Because fruits and vegetables found in most supermarkets and many produce stands are shipped from long distances, they are harvested before they ripen and are therefore missing a portion of these vital life chemicals. Even so, you will receive far more nutrition from store bought produce than from processed foods, as all raw fruits and vegetables contain enzymes and antioxidants. Under no circumstances can processed foods make this claim.

While scientific research continues to unravel the protective role of phytochemicals against heart disease and cancer, we already know that these vital life chemicals are natural components of a plant's defense system. As plants are protected against the sun's harmful ultraviolet rays, humans who eat a diet high in plant food are also protected.

Until I began drinking carrot juice, my skin burned easily when exposed to the sun. I can now spend hours in the sun without suffering sunburn. Incidentally, I never use sunscreens; my carrot juice and other raw foods protect me.

Phytochemicals provide each body cell with the enzymes it needs for growth, digestion, heartbeat, blood pressure, elimination, and so on. The only foods which contain enzymes are raw or slightly steamed foods. According to doctors of natural health, enzymes begin to suffer harm at 107 degrees Fahrenheit and are destroyed at temperatures above 118 degrees.

A person is born with an "enzyme bank," but if that person fails to make regular deposits to that bank by eating foods which contain enzymes, his body functions will overdraw his bank account of enzymes. Thus, he will stand a great chance of experiencing digestive problems, constipation, diarrhea, spastic colon, candidiasis, heart disease, high blood pressure, gallstones, kidney stones, diabetes, anemia, obesity, headaches, restlessness, tumors, cancer, and a multitude of other unwanted ailments.

Phytochemicals supply the body with antioxidants in the form of Vitamins A (beta carotene,) C, and E, which neutralize the cell damaging free radicals formed in our bodies every day. I am convinced that the body assimilates phytochemicals from food much more efficiently than it assimilates vitamins and minerals in pill form.

I am not opposed to taking vitamins if there is a need to do so; however, I contend that God created plants for humans to eat, and within these plants, He placed all the nutrition needed for the human body. The argument of those who promote vitamin pills is that a person would have to eat several pounds of vegetables per day in order to get the quantity of vitamins and minerals equal to the content of a few pills. This may be true; however, the body does not assimilate a pill the way that God designed it to assimilate food. As raw, unprocessed foods enter the body, they enhance the body to produce the necessary vitamins and minerals needed for its many functions.

And God said, Behold, I have given you every herb bearing seed, which is upon the face of all the earth, and every tree, in the which is the fruit of a tree yielding seed; to you it shall be for meat. Gen. 1:29

4

Are You Acid Or Alkaline?

Another thing we need to consider is that the body needs a balance of alkaline forming foods as well as acid forming foods. Doctors of alternative medicine recommend a diet high in alkaline forming foods for those who are ill. Viruses and diseases thrive in an acid environment, but they cannot tolerate an alkaline environment. If this theory works to make sick people well, why won't it work to keep healthy people healthy?

Your pH level determines whether you are acid or alkaline. PH, a symbol for the degree of acidity or alkalinity of a solution, is the method of measuring the *hydrogen power* of a solution. This may be done by a blood or saliva test. The pH of pure water is 7.0, which is neutral. Any reading below 7.0 is acid, while any reading above 7.0 is alkaline. It is not difficult for the average American to get plenty of acid in the diet, but one usually has to make a special effort to eat enough alkaline forming foods.

Some of the most common acid forming foods are butter, catsup, cheeses, cocoa, coffee, cornstarch, eggs, fish, flour products, canned foods, dried coconut, meat, milk, mustard, pasta, poultry, sauerkraut, shellfish, soft drinks, sugar, and tea.

Some alkaline forming foods are almonds, apricots, avocados, Brazil nuts, buckwheat, corn, dates, fresh coconut, fresh fruits, honey, lemons, maple syrup, melons, millet, oranges, raisins, most fresh vegetables, and soured dairy products.

On the following pages, we will examine some foods which are familiar to you along with other foods not common to the American diet. You must be the one to decide which foods you will eat and which ones you will avoid.

To Eat Or Not To Eat?

Butter - Buy organic butter if at all possible. Eat it in moderation as it is high in fat - but no higher than margarine. Keep in mind that butter is a whole food, whereas margarine is not. The body can process whole foods much easier than it can process chemical compounds. Butter is mentioned favorably in the Bible.

Canned Foods - I once heard a doctor ask, "Why buy and prepare something that someone else has cooked? Why not cook it yourself so you'll know exactly what's in it?"

The body needs a proper balance of sodium and potassium. God put this balance in whole foods. Approximately four ounces of peas fresh from the garden contain 316 mg of potassium and 2 mg of sodium. Put these peas through the canning process and you have 236 mg of sodium and 96 mg of potassium, no digestive enzymes, and possibly 20% of the original nutritional value.

Chips - Most chips are fried and contain harmful additives and preservatives. If you must include chips in your diet, read the ingredients carefully and purchase baked chips without oils. You may find these at a health food store and in a few grocery stores.

Chocolate - Contains a lot of fat and sugar; leads to compulsive eating. Contains only a small amount of caffeine but a large amount of theobromine, a strong stimulant. A mood altering substance that can have strong effects on body and mind and can surely be addictive.

Coffee - The strongest of all caffeine sources. Decaffeinated coffee still contains small amounts of caffeine as well as other active substances present in coffee beans that can be irritating to the nervous, gastrointestinal, and urinary systems.

Eggs - Eggs are a whole food. Don't be afraid to eat them. If possible, buy fresh eggs from a farmer who has free roaming hens. Avoid grocery store eggs that have been in the cooler for days and perhaps weeks. These eggs have been laid by hens crammed into cramped cages. How can chickens under such stress lay healthful eggs? If you have no other source, buy your eggs from a health food store that sells organic eggs laid by free roaming hens.

Fresh Fruits and Vegetables - The best plan is to grow them yourself, but most of us find that impossible. Second best is to buy them as fresh as possible. If there are times that you simply cannot buy them fresh, buy them frozen - never canned. Try to find a reliable produce stand which buys from local farmers on a regular basis. If you cannot buy organic, try one of the following methods to soak away the pesticides.

1. Add one cup of freshly extracted lemon juice to three gallons of water and soak ten minutes. Rinse thoroughly and soak in clear water another ten minutes.

2. Wash and scrub produce with hydrogen peroxide full strength; then soak in clear water for ten minutes.

3. Add one cup of vinegar to three gallons of water. Soak your produce in this solution ten minutes, rinse, and then soak another ten minutes in clear water.

It is very important to buy your fruits fresh, as it is difficult to find frozen fruits that do not contain sugar and harmful preservatives. Eat the peelings and the seeds when you can. Both grape seeds and apple seeds are high in antioxidants. Of course, you wouldn't eat orange or grapefruit peelings.

Fried Foods - Never eat fried foods. Fats are altered by high temperatures and even more so when used repeatedly. They undergo a chemical change and form new harmful compounds such as benzene. Benzene is a clear, flammable, poisonous aromatic liquid used in plastics, paints, dyes, insecticides, and detergents. Would you eat these substances?

Grains - Whole grains should be a part of your daily diet. Some suggestions are brown rice, quinoa, millet, amaranth, barley, and corn. Whole grain rice is often referred to as *brown rice*. It is more healthful than white rice, as it still contains the bran (outer layer) of the grain, which provides a large proportion of many vitamins and minerals, especially B vitamins.

Herbs and Spices - Use these for seasoning your foods, as opposed to using fats and oils. Oregano, basil, thyme, chives, garlic, tarragon, and parsley are some of my favorites for seasoning vegetables, grains, and legumes. Cinnamon and ginger make excellent flavorings for fruit dishes and sweet breads. Herbs have medicinal value in addition to being tasty.

Honey - Raw, unheated - preferably Tupelo. The body absorbs it rather slowly in comparison to sugar. It has its own nutrients used to digest itself, whereas refined sugar does not. Honey is mentioned favorably in the Bible.

Instant foods - instant potatoes, instant oatmeal, etc. - Avoid these at all times. Not only do they contain harmful preservatives; their nutrients have been destroyed by extensive processing.

Legumes - These should be a part of your daily diet. Peas and beans complement the protein in grains. A legume combined with a grain raises the protein content of a meal and increases its nutritional value. Blackeye peas, navy beans, lentils, black beans, garbanzo beans, red beans, split peas, lima beans, butterbeans, and all other legumes are very nutritious.

Margarine - According to the label, it is made from polyunsaturated oil. Read the ingredients. It is an emulsion of fats, emulsifying agents, sodium benzoate, artificial coloring, flavors, and vitamins. On most margarine, you will see the phrase "partially hydrogenated oils," meaning that the oil is no longer polyunsaturated! In essence, margarine is highly processed. Butter is a much better choice.

Milk - Contrary to what we were taught in school, milk is not the best source of calcium. Soybeans, dried beans, walnuts, sunflower seeds, and green vegetables provide plenty of calcium for the body without adverse effects. Milk coats the intestines with a film-like, mucous substance, and the mucous spreads inside the body, even into the respiratory system. Eliminating milk from the diet has been known to relieve sinus problems.

Raw, unprocessed milk contains the enzyme lipase which God placed there to digest and assimilate the fat. Pasteurization destroys this enzyme. Homogenization does even more damage by separating the fat molecules so the cream doesn't stay on top. One molecule may become 20, 50, 100, or more smaller pieces, requiring multiple amounts of enzymes and digestive juices.

Unless you are allergic to dairy products or have a condition such as candidiasis, you may use buttermilk and some pasteurized milk for cooking. Should you choose not to use dairy products, try rice milk or oat milk.

Nuts - Contain a large amount of high quality protein and essential fatty acids. Eat them raw and unsalted. The ideal way to buy nuts is in the hull. It is time consuming to crack and shell them, but you will have a fresher, more healthful product. If you do buy them shelled, be sure they are raw and contain no preservatives, never cooked or salted.

Olive Oil - Buy pure, cold-pressed (unheated) extra virgin olive oil. It is hard to find, but it is the safest oil to use. It has been reported that olive oil can actually lower blood cholesterol.

Processed sandwich meat, hot dogs, etc. - Stay away from the "deli" area of the grocery store. Never buy sausage meat, bacon, pepperoni, etc. You have no way of knowing the ingredients or how they were prepared. Pork products and processed sandwich meat contains nitrates and/or nitrites. All hot dogs contain these cancer forming chemicals as well as harmful dyes. Hot dogs are at least 70% trash - stuff you would throw in the garbage if it were in your kitchen in its true form. Does it make any sense to pay big bucks for someone else's garbage and contaminate your body with it? Even worse is to contaminate the little bodies of your precious children. A study at University of Southern California revealed that children who eat three hot dogs per week have nine times the risk of leukemia as children who do not eat hot dogs. According to the laws of math, if a child eats one hot dog per week, he has three times the risk of leukemia as children who do not eat hot dogs.

Salt - You may be surprised to find that salt is frequently used in my recipes. The Bible speaks favorably of salt as a seasoning, so why should I have a problem with it? Yet, it is next to impossible to find natural salt today.

The list of ingredients on a box of table salt on the grocery store shelf reads, "salt, calcium silicate, dextrose, and potassium oxide." Many brands of sea salt in health food stores list the same ingredients! Look for solar sea salt labeled "Sun dried only. Not kiln dried. Nothing added or removed." If you have salt and pepper mills, you might use rock salt. Be sure to buy a brand recommended for table use. Some rock salt is to be used only for melting snow or making ice cream. In any case, use salt sparingly. Salt is a mineral and needs to be balanced with other minerals, especially potassium. Many foods contain sufficient amounts of natural salt, celery being a good example of this. You can also season your foods with herbs or liquid aminos and avoid the consequences of too much salt.

Seeds - Better raw and unprocessed. They contain less fat than nuts do and are high in protein.

Sugar - Refined sugar is a simple carbohydrate, stripped of all nutrients, consisting solely of empty calories. Vitamins, minerals, and protein are necessary for the metabolism of sugar. Because sugar cannot supply these nutrients, they are pulled from the bones and tissues of the body in order to metabolize the sugar. The body digests sugar cane (a whole food) at one calorie per minute; it digests white sugar at ten calories per minute! Sugar cane has the nutrients needed for digestion. Unfortunately, these nutrients are processed out by the time it becomes white sugar.

Soft Drinks - They contain carbon dioxide as well as phosphoric acid made by treating phosphorus with sulfuric acid. They also contain an enormous amount of sugar. Diet drinks? Not on your life! Aspartame has been linked with seizures. I urge you <u>never</u> to drink soft drinks; however, if you are going to do so anyway, please drink the sugar filled ones as opposed to the diet drinks. As harmful as they are, they are the lesser of the two evils.

Tea - As a rule, I do not recommend teas which contain caffeine. Many herbal teas do not contain caffeine. Read the labels and make sure you are getting a caffeine free tea.

Kitchen Aids - Helpful Or Harmful?

Aluminum Cookware - Aluminum accumulates in the body. Studies have shown high levels of aluminum in the body to be linked with brain damage and Alzheimer's.

Try this experiment: Place a tarnished silver object in a clean aluminum pan and cover it with approximately 1 1/2 inches of water. Add one teaspoon baking soda to the water and boil it five minutes. The aluminum will dissolve as ions. Silver ions in the sulfide will be redeposited on the surface of the object. The baking soda will serve as an inert electrolyte. Use tongs to remove the object and buff it with a clean cloth. Do the same experiment with another tarnished silver object using a stainless steel pan. Stainless steel will not dissolve and combine with the silver. Neither will it combine with food cooked in it.

If you are presently using aluminum cookware, please replace it with stainless steel or glass cookware as soon as possible. In the meantime, line your aluminum baking dishes with wax paper. Butter the wax paper and pour your cake mixtures, bread mixtures, etc. onto the buttered wax paper for baking.

Blender - Used to puree vegetables, chop nuts, blend ingredients for cream soups, etc.

Bread Maker - A time saver for making homemade bread.

Corningware, Glassware - Serviceable and harmless.

Iron Cookware - Time-tested and almost universally considered to be healthful and safe. Keep the utensils clean and smooth. Do not leave water or acid foods standing in the skillets. This will cause the utensils to rust and discolor the food.

Juicer - I have two - the citrus juicer and the regular juice extractor. Juices have many health benefits. Take the time to juice <u>fresh</u> fruits and vegetables so you will reap the benefits of enzymes in addition to raising your alkaline level.

Microwave - The microwave is a little box of radiation. The argument is, "It is low-energy, non-ionizing radiation." Think about it. Do you really want a constant source of low-level radiation in your home? Incidentally, radiation <u>does</u> leak out. All radiation is harmful to the body. You cannot smell, taste, or feel it as it accumulates in the body. There is no dose of radiation so low that the risk is zero. Any amount of cooking destroys enzymes as well as some of the nutrients in food. Radiation destroys them quicker and more severely. Food cells, which will become part of your body cells, are drastically changed as the radiation heats from the inside as opposed to the conventional method which begins at the outside of the food and moves toward the middle. I do not have a microwave in my home.

Mixer - Very helpful in making desserts, pancakes, muffins, and certain kinds of bread. If you do not have an electric mixer, an egg beater may be used.

Salad Shooter - A time saving device for making salads, grating coconut, cheese, etc.

Sifter or wire strainer - Sift whole grain flour and cornmeal before measuring.

Stainless Steel Cookware - Serviceable and harmless; does not combine with foods cooked in it.

Steamer - Steamed vegetables are delicious and nutritious!

Tea Maker - Known as a coffee maker to most people but used exclusively in my home to make herbal teas.

Chapter 2

BEGIN WITH

BREAKFAST

That's my cup o' tea

Breakfast

My recommendation is that you always eat breakfast. If you simply do not care for food that early in the morning, force yourself to at least eat a piece of fruit and drink a glass of juice. Proper foods nourish the brain as well as the body and provide much needed energy to begin the day.

If you feel that you do not have time to eat breakfast, get up a few minutes earlier. Several years ago, my husband and I heard an interesting news report. A group of doctors had determined that the mind tends to be more alert between the hours of 8:00 a.m. and 11:00 a.m. than at any other time during the day. Statistics showed that those who ate breakfast were more alert and had a higher energy level throughout the day than those who did not eat breakfast.

I never recommend eating meat for breakfast. Your body has undergone the assimilation cycle during your sleeping hours and is now in the elimination cycle. Allow your body to digest juices, raw fruits, nuts, and grain products during the early hours of the day. Schedules will vary for those who work shifts, but as often as possible, get up at the same time every day, eat your meals at the same time, exercise at the same time, and go to bed at the same time.

One more thing about breakfast: If you are one who wants something filling but do not care to eat the traditional breakfast foods morning after morning, why not have leftovers from the night before? There's nothing wrong with that - just try to avoid meat until later in the day.

Oatmeal

Use 100% rolled oats and cook five to ten minutes. Avoid instant oatmeal or any oatmeal that has other ingredients such as fruit and other flavors added. Sweeten your oatmeal with honey, barley malt, or stevia.

Nuts

Make yourself a side dish with banana and walnuts or choose your own favorite fruit and nuts. Just be sure your fruit is fresh (never canned) and your nuts should be raw and unprocessed.

Toast

A slice of toast made from whole grain bread is nutritious. Use butter on your toast. If you like jelly with your toast, buy one of the fruit products containing no sugar. Keep in mind that this is a processed fruit - no longer alkaline, but acid. It is okay once in a while, but don't eat it often.

French Toast

2 eggs
1 cup oat milk or rice milk
1/4 teaspoon nutmeg
1/2 tsp. vanilla extract
6 slices whole grain bread
cinnamon

Mix eggs, milk, and vanilla together. Dip bread in mixture, then place on a buttered grill or skillet. Sprinkle with cinnamon and cook on medium heat until golden brown. Serve with pure maple syrup or rice syrup. Serves two to three people.

Pancakes

Pancakes are a delicious breakfast food. You can use whole wheat flour, barley flour, or spelt flour. Whole milk works well; however, if you prefer to use a grain milk such as rice milk, oat milk, or soy milk, add 1/4 teaspoon Xanthan gum to each cup of flour. This adds consistency to the batter.

Pancakes # 1

1 cup flour
2 teaspoons baking powder
1/2 teaspoon salt
2 Tablespoons olive oil
1 cup milk (or 1/2 cup buttermilk + 1/2 cup water)
If using grain milk, add 1/4 teaspoon Xanthan gum

Butter a skillet or grill, place on burner, and turn heat to medium high. Mix all ingredients together. Beat one minute on medium speed. Texture should be smooth but not runny. Pour onto hot grill or skillet. The pancakes will need to be flipped within one to two minutes. Cook thoroughly on both sides and serve hot. Serves two hungry or three light eaters.

Pancakes # 2

1 cup flour
2 teaspoons baking soda
1/2 teaspoon salt
2 Tablespoons olive oil
1 Tablespoon honey
1 cup milk (or 1/2 cup buttermilk + 1/2 cup water)
If using grain milk, add 1/4 teaspoon Xanthan gum

Follow cooking instructions above for Pancakes # 1

Yogurt Pancakes

1 cup flour
2 teaspoons baking powder
1/2 teaspoon salt
2 Tablespoons olive oil

1 egg
1/2 cup yogurt
1/4 cup water

Follow cooking instructions for Pancakes # 1 on previous page.

Yellow Corn Grits

2 1/2 cups water
2/3 cup yellow corn grits
1/2 teaspoon salt
2 teaspoons liquid aminos
(It is okay to use white grits; just don't use instant grits!)

Pour water into saucepan and set burner on medium-high. Add salt, liquid aminos, then grits. Boil three to five minutes, stirring constantly. Grits will thicken as you stir.

For variety, stir in a whole raw egg. Stir rapidly, as it cooks quickly - in about thirty seconds. Until you are comfortable working with raw eggs, you may need to beat the egg before adding it to your grits. Add a little extra salt from your salt shaker for the egg. For added color and to enhance the taste, sprinkle with a little parsley. Serves three or four.

Millet

Millet is a whole grain with much nutritional value. Follow directions on the package. Add a 1/2 teaspoon salt and 2 teaspoons liquid aminos to 2/3 cup millet. You might even try adding a few herbs to your millet - oregano is good. May be eaten alone or with fruit, eggs and other breakfast foods.

Other Suggestions for Breakfast

If you feel that you must eat cereal, select one high in whole grains and relatively low in sweeteners. Even though cereal at its best is a processed food, you can carefully read the ingredients and choose one which does not contain sugar or any artificial sweetener such as aspartame. Amaranth flakes, bran flakes, or spelt flakes are an excellent choice. Sprinkle with lecithin granules or add a little honey or rice syrup. Serve with oat milk, rice milk, or multi grain milk.

I have yet to find a cereal on the grocery store shelves which meets the above requirements. It may be necessary to purchase your cereals from a health food store. Even so, eat in moderation. As healthful as your cereal may be, it is a processed food containing no enzymes.

Breakfast Drinks

If you like a hot drink for breakfast, experiment with herbal teas until you find one you really like. My favorite morning teas are Rose Hips and Red Raspberry. Your body does not need caffeine; you will get a more healthful boost from freshly extracted juice. If you are a hot chocolate drinker, try hot carob sweetened with honey or stevia.

An excellent way to begin your day is to drink six to eight ounces of freshly extracted carrot juice. If at all possible, use organic carrots. They are very sweet tasting. If you have a juicer, make your own. Discard the fiber unless you plan to use it within a day or two to thicken soup. If you have not yet purchased a juicer or if you simply do not have the time to juice, the next best plan is to buy freeze dried carrot juice and mix with water.

Water is always the best drink for any meal - breakfast included.

Chapter 3

LET'S BAKE

BREAD

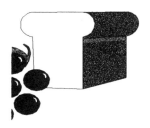

Give us this day our daily bread. Matthew 6:11

Bread

Always use whole grain flour or meal; never use white bleached flour. Sift your flour or meal. Bake your bread in stainless steel, iron, or glass ovenware. If you do not have stainless steel muffin pans, place disposable muffin cups in your aluminum or coated muffin pans. Read the information on page 12 regarding aluminum cookware.

If you look at a bag of white flour on the grocery shelf, you will most likely see the word "enriched." How is it enriched? Why is it enriched?

First of all, the flour was milled. Then it was refined and often bleached. Essential vitamins and minerals were lost in significant quantities. White flour contains less than 1/3 pyridoxine and folic acid and less than 1/2 of the pantothenic acid found in whole wheat flour. It contains only 13% of the chromium, 9% of the manganese, 19% of the iron, and about 14% of the vitamin E found in whole wheat flour. Thus, it is required by law to be "enriched." However, the "enriching" process replaces only a *small fraction* of the nutrients which have been taken away in the refining process.

Doctors of natural health have determined that refined foods contribute greatly to tooth decay. They also clog the colon as they do not contain enough fiber to digest them properly.

Never use pancake mixes, cornbread mixes, biscuit mixes, etc. These are even more processed than white flour. The more processed your ingredients, the fewer nutrients your bread will contain. Use whole grains. You will find that breads made from refined flour do not have the good rich texture of those made from whole grains.

Using A Bread Machine

If you use a bread machine for the recipes which call for kneading, follow the directions that came with your bread machine. First add the salt, oil, and honey to the warm water. Then carefully pour the flour and gluten over these ingredients. Make a small dent in the center of the flour to pour the yeast. This is to prevent the yeast from touching the salt or the water too soon. Should this happen, the bread will begin to rise too quickly and will fall before the process is finished. Choose a "whole wheat" setting. This will take approximately four hours, and you will not need to knead!

Bread Without A Bread Machine

Dissolve regular yeast in warm water (warm but not hot to the touch of the hand) by stirring approximately one minute. Add salt and liquid ingredients such as honey and oil. Let this mixture stand while you place the flour, gluten, and all other dry ingredients into another bowl. Always sift flour before measuring. Now pour the liquid ingredients over the dry ingredients gradually, stirring well. It helps to make a crevice in the middle of the dry ingredients and pour the liquid mixture into it, stirring from the middle. After mixing thoroughly, place in a buttered bowl, cover with a soft clean cloth and let stand 15 minutes. The dough will begin to rise. Stir down and knead (mix and work into a pliable mass by folding over, pressing, and squeezing with the hands) five minutes on a floured board. Let rise 45 minutes (until double in size) in a buttered, covered bowl in a warm place. Knead another five minutes, place in a well buttered, average size (9"x5"x3") loaf pan, cover and let rise another 45 minutes. Remove cover and bake 45-50 minutes at 350 degrees.

Both Spelt Bread and Whole Wheat Bread # 1 may be made either with or without the use of a bread machine. Follow instructions on page 22.

Spelt Bread

2 1/2 cups spelt flour
3 Tablespoons gluten
1 1/4 cup warm water
1 Tablespoon olive oil

2 Tablespoons honey
1 teaspoon salt
1 teaspoon baking soda
1 1/2 teaspoon dry yeast
(one package regular)

Whole Wheat Bread #1

2 1/2 cups whole wheat flour
2 Tablespoons gluten
1 1/4 cup warm water
1 Tablespoon olive oil

2 Tablespoons honey
1/2 teaspoon salt
1 1/2 teaspoon dry yeast
(one package regular)

Whole Wheat Bread # 2

1 cup warm water
1 Tablespoon dry yeast
(two packages regular)
1 Tablespoon honey

1 Tablespoon molasses
1 teaspoon salt
3 cups whole wheat flour
1 teaspoon lecithin granules

Dissolve yeast in warm water. Add honey, molasses, salt, and 1 cup flour. Mix thoroughly with a spoon and let stand 10 minutes. Stir down and let stand 15 minutes. Add lecithin and 2 cups flour. Knead 3 minutes. Shape into loaf and place in buttered 9"x5"x3" loaf pan. Cover and let rise 45 minutes in a warm place. Remove cover and bake 45 minutes at 350 degrees.

Multi-Grain Bread

1 1/4 cups warm water
2 Tablespoons honey
2 Tablespoons olive oil
1 teaspoon salt
3 Tablespoons gluten
1 1/2 teaspoons (one package regular) dry yeast

1 1/2 cups whole wheat flour
1/4 cup oatmeal
1/4 cup corn meal
1/4 cup flax seed
1/4 cup sunflower seeds

Use your blender to blend oatmeal, flax seed, and sunflower seeds until they become a coarse flour. Follow mixing and baking instructions on page 22 for either kneading by hand or using a bread machine. Consider the oatmeal, corn meal, flax seed, and sunflower seeds a part of the flour mixture.

Whole Wheat Rolls

1 Tablespoon dry yeast
2 cups warm water
2 teaspoons salt
1 teaspoon lecithin (optional)

1/4 cup butter
2 beaten eggs
1/3 cup honey
6 cups whole wheat flour

Dissolve yeast in warm water. Cream together butter, eggs, and honey. Add this mixture to the yeast and warm water. Mix well. Work in the salt and flour. Knead dough about 5 minutes. Put in a buttered bowl, cover and let rise in a warm place about 45 minutes or until double in size. Punch down and form small balls approximately one inch in diameter. Place the balls on a buttered baking sheet about 3 inches apart. Cover and let rise again 30 to 45 minutes until light and doubled. Remove cover and bake 12 to 15 minutes at 400 degrees. Makes about five dozen rolls. Use some now and freeze some for later use.

Yeast Biscuits

1/2 cup warm water
1 Tablespoon regular yeast
  (2 packages)
1 Tablespoon honey
1 teaspoon salt

2 1/2 cups whole wheat flour
5 Tablespoons olive oil
1/2 cup warm buttermilk
  (warm, not hot to the touch)

Dissolve yeast by stirring it into the warm water. Add honey and salt. Let the mixture set five minutes. Sift the flour into another bowl in the meantime and make a large crevice in the middle of the flour. Now add the olive oil and the buttermilk to the warm water mixture. Stir lightly. Stirring from the center, slowly pour the liquid ingredients into the crevice of the flour, bringing the flour a little at the time into the mixture. After the liquid and dry ingredients are thoroughly mixed, knead lightly. Form into about one dozen biscuits and place on a buttered baking sheet or in a muffin pan. Let them rise 30 minutes. If they rise in muffin tins, they will easily rise upward. If they rise on a baking sheet, they will rise out and up. Bake 25 minutes at 400 degrees.

Baking Powder Biscuits

2 cups whole wheat flour
1 teaspoon salt
4 teaspoons baking powder

1 cup buttermilk
1/4 cup olive oil
1/2 teaspoon Xanthan gum

Sift flour. Make a large crevice in the middle. Pour the baking powder, salt, and gluten into the crevice. Now pour the olive oil into the crevice. Begin stirring from the center of the crevice, bringing the flour a little at the time into the mixture. While stirring, slowly add the buttermilk. Use a spoon to stir until thoroughly mixed, then knead lightly with the hands. Form into biscuits and place on a buttered baking sheet or iron griddle. Bake 15 minutes at 450 degrees. Makes about 7-8.

Barley Muffins

1 cup barley flour, sifted	1 egg (beaten)
2 teaspoons baking powder	2 Tablespoons olive oil
1/2 teaspoon salt	1/2 cup water

Butter a muffin pan or use disposable muffin holders. Sift the flour into a bowl and make a large crevice in the middle. Put the baking powder, salt, olive oil, and egg into the hole. Stir from the center, bringing the flour a little at the time into the mixture. While stirring, add the water slowly. Stir until all the flour is a part of the mixture. Pour into a buttered muffin pan or use disposable muffin cups. Bake 15 to 20 minutes at 425 degrees. Makes six large muffins or as many as twelve small ones.

If you prefer, you can bake the barley biscuits on a buttered stainless steel cookie sheet. Just spoon them out in 11 or 12 small portions leaving a little space between them. They will be smaller and flatter than those baked in a muffin pan.

Blueberry Muffins

1 egg	1 3/4 cups whole wheat flour
3/4 cup milk	1 1/2 teaspoon baking soda
2 Tablespoons olive oil	1/4 teaspoon salt
1/4 cup honey	1 cup fresh or frozen blueberries (drain if you use frozen ones)

Butter a muffin pan or use disposable muffin holders. Mix liquid ingredients, then add dry ingredients and mix thoroughly on medium speed. Fold in blueberries. Fill muffin tins 1/2 full. Bake 30 minutes at 325 degrees. Makes 10-12 muffins.

Bran Muffins # 1

2 eggs, beaten
2 Tablespoon olive oil
1/2 cup honey
1 cup apple juice
(unsweetened)

1 cup whole wheat flour
1 teaspoon baking soda
1/4 teaspoon salt
1 cup wheat bran or rice bran

Butter a muffin pan or use disposable muffin holders. Beat on low speed the eggs, olive oil, honey, and apple juice. In another bowl, stir together all dry ingredients. Combine all ingredients and beat on medium speed until thoroughly mixed. Fill muffin tins 1/2 full. Bake 30 minutes at 325 degrees. Makes about one dozen muffins.

Bran Muffins # 2

1 cup wheat bran or rice bran
1 cup whole wheat flour
1 1/4 teaspoon baking soda
1/4 teaspoon salt
1/4 teaspoon cinnamon (optional)

1/2 cup butter
1/2 cup honey
2 eggs, beaten
1 cup buttermilk

Follow instructions for Bran Muffins #1, considering the cinnamon as one of the dry ingredients.

For Bran Muffin Variety:

To add flavor and variety to your bran muffins, include one of the following:

1/2 cup raisins and/or sunflower seeds
1 cup finely chopped apples
1 mashed ripe banana
1 cup fresh or frozen blueberries
Sprinkle nutmeg or cinnamon as desired

Cornbread

1 1/2 cup yellow cornmeal (white may be used if preferred)
1/2 cup whole wheat flour   1/4 cup olive oil
4 teaspoons baking powder   2 eggs
1 teaspoon salt   1 1/2 cups milk or buttermilk

Preheat oven to 400 degrees. Butter a 9" square or round baking dish. Sift cornmeal and flour before measuring. In medium bowl sift together all dry ingredients. In small bowl beat together eggs, oil, and milk. Now add this mixture to the dry ingredients and beat all until completely moistened. Spread batter evenly into a buttered 9" square or round baking dish, place in preheated oven, and bake 35 minutes or until golden brown at 400 degrees.

If you prefer to make corn muffins, fill 10-12 muffin pans half full. Bake muffins 20 minutes in preheated oven at 425 degrees.

Millet Bread

2 eggs   2 cups millet flour
1/4 cup olive oil   4 teaspoons baking soda
1/4 cup honey   1 teaspoon salt
1 1/2 cups buttermilk (Substitute 1 cup rice milk
                        or oat milk if desired)

Preheat oven to 325 degrees. Butter a 9" square or round baking dish. Sift millet flour before measuring. Sift together with other dry ingredients after measuring. In small bowl beat together eggs, oil, and milk. Add this mixture to the dry ingredients and beat until completely moistened. Spread batter evenly into a buttered 9" square or round baking dish, place in preheated oven, and bake 35 minutes or until golden brown at 325 degrees.

The following sweetbreads may also be made as muffins. Each recipe will make approximately 12-15 regular size muffins.

Cranberry Bread

2 cups whole wheat flour, sifted
1 1/2 teaspoon baking powder
1 teaspoon baking soda
3/4 cup apple juice or orange juice
1 cup cranberries, chopped

1 egg
1/2 cup butter
1/2 cup honey

Sift flour, baking powder, and baking soda together and set aside. In another bowl, slightly beat the egg, butter and honey. Add orange juice to liquid mixture and stir. Now add dry ingredients. Beat at medium speed until all ingredients are mixed well. Add cranberries and stir until thoroughly mixed. Pour into a buttered 9"x5"x3" loaf pan and bake one hour and 10 minutes at 325 degrees. Cool 20 minutes before slicing.

Honey Nut Bread

2 1/2 cups whole wheat flour, sifted
2 teaspoons baking powder
1/2 teaspoon baking soda
3/4 cup walnuts, chopped

1 egg, beaten
1/2 cup butter
3/4 cup honey
3/4 cup orange juice

Sift flour, baking powder, and baking soda together and set aside. In another bowl, slightly beat the egg, butter and honey. Add orange juice to liquid mixture and stir. Now add dry ingredients and beat at medium speed until thoroughly mixed. Add walnuts and stir thoroughly. Pour into a buttered 9x5x3 loaf pan and bake one hour and 10 minutes at 325 degrees. Cool 20 minutes before slicing.

Banana Bread

1/2 cup butter	1 teaspoon baking soda
1/2 cup honey	1 teaspoon salt
2 eggs	1 3/4 cups whole wheat flour
2 large bananas	1/2 cup broken walnut pieces

Preheat oven to 325 degrees. Butter an average size (4"x8") loaf pan. Sift flour before measuring, then place in a medium bowl and use a fork to stir baking soda and salt into the flour. In a large bowl mix together butter, honey, and eggs. Mash bananas with a fork, then beat into the mixture. Add dry ingredients gradually, continuing to mix. Then stir in broken walnut pieces. Pour into a buttered loaf pan and bake approximately 1 hour, 10 minutes at 325 degrees. Check after one hour by inserting a toothpick in the center. If the toothpick comes out clean, the bread is done.

Zucchini Bread

2 eggs	1/2 teaspoon baking powder
1/2 cup honey	1/4 teaspoon ground ginger
1/2 cup olive oil	1 1/2 cups whole wheat flour
1/2 teaspoon salt	1 zucchini squash, grated
1/2 teaspoon baking soda	1/2 cup walnut pieces

Preheat oven to 325 degrees. Butter a 9" square pan. Grate a zucchini squash. The zucchini should be about 1 1/2 cups, loosely packed. Sift flour before measuring. Beat eggs, honey, and oil together in a large bowl. Stir in dry ingredients and zucchini. Add broken walnuts and stir until thoroughly mixed. Bake in a buttered 9" square pan for one hour at 325 degrees.

Mary's Bible Bread (2 loaves)
Find the dry ingredients in Ezekiel 4:9

1 cup whole wheat flour	1 1/2 cup warm water
1/2 cup barley flour	1 Tablespoon dry yeast
1/2 cup soy flour	1 teaspoon salt
1/4 cup lentils (raw, blended)	2 Tablespoons honey
1/4 cup millet	2 Tablespoons olive oil
1/2 cup fitches (spelt)	3 Tablespoons gluten

Dissolve yeast in warm water. Add salt, honey, molasses and oil. Mix with a spoon. You will have three cups of dry ingredients. Sift them together, add gradually to the liquids, and continue to stir. When thoroughly mixed, knead 5 minutes. Dough will be smooth and elastic. Put in buttered bowl and cover. Let rise 45 minutes or until double in size. Punch down. Place in a buttered 9"x5"x3" loaf pan. Cover and let rise another 45 minutes. Remove cover, spread butter over the top for a soft crust, and bake 55 minutes at 350 degrees.

Option: Make **Mary's Bible Bread** using the same measures of all ingredients with two exceptions. Omit the warm water and yeast. Add 2 Tablespoons baking soda and 1 1/2 cup buttermilk. Do not knead. Pour into a 9" square buttered pan and bake at 350 for 45 to 50 minutes.

Mary's Garlic Spread For Bread

1/2 cup (1 stick) melted butter

1 teaspoon oregano	1/2 teaspoon thyme
1 teaspoon garlic	1 teaspoon basil

Stir all ingredients together. Spread evenly on several slices of bread. You will have enough of the mixture for 14-16 slices. May be refrigerated for later use.

Nutri-Nut Bread

1/2 cup butter	1/4 cup chopped cashews
3 eggs	1/3 cup bran
3/4 cup honey	1/4 cup flax seeds
1/4 cup molasses	2 cups whole wheat flour
1 cup orange juice	1/4 cup sunflower seeds
1 cup grated carrots	1/4 cup chopped walnuts
1/2 teaspoon salt	1/2 cup raisins
2 teaspoons baking soda	2 T. lecithin granules

Preheat oven to 300 degrees. Butter a 9" square baking pan. Sift flour before measuring. Blend (in blender) the flax seed until it becomes as flour. In a large bowl mix together butter, eggs, honey, molasses, and juice. Add salt, baking soda, blended flax seed, bran, and lecithin. Beat with mixer. Add the flour and beat well. Stir in the carrots, cashews, sunflower seeds, walnuts, and raisins. Pour into a 9" square baking pan. Bake one hour and 15 minutes at 300 degrees.

Broad Bread Hints

Try the preceding recipes. Think about what you might add to make each one more tasty. For instance, imagine what spelt bread would taste like with your favorite nuts or seeds. Create your own recipes accordingly.

Unfortunately, most of us have used bread mixes and white flour so long, we find it difficult to work with whole grains. If you have this problem, buy a bag of unbleached white flour and make bread a few times. Use in combination with whole grains, each time decreasing the portion of unbleached white until you are totally using whole grains. Most health food stores carry whole wheat pastry flour which may be preferred over regular whole wheat flour for making cakes and breads.

Chapter 4

SUPER

SALADS

And God said, Let the earth bring forth grass, the herb yielding seed, and the fruit tree yielding fruit after his kind, whose seed is in itself upon the earth, and it was so. Genesis 1:11

Vegetable Salad

Ideally, a large vegetable salad made of six or seven different vegetables should be eaten at least once each day. Two or three times per day would not be too much. I cannot overemphasize the value of raw vegetables.

There is no steadfast rule as to how to make a salad. Use whatever you have on hand. Here are some suggestions. Red leaf or green leaf lettuce, spinach, broccoli, kale, carrots, cucumber, tomatoes, cauliflower, and the list goes on. If you like raw onions and celery, these may also be added. Sprinkle with your favorite herbs. Thyme, basil, parsley, and oregano are tasty. Try to eat your salad without dressing. If you simply must have a dressing on your salad, use an olive oil and vinegar dressing. Add some herbs to the mixture. Liquid aminos is very tasty on salad. Some health food stores carry a tofu based salad dressing. Whatever dressing you use, try to cut back and eat less of it until you are eating your salad plain. Savor the flavor of fresh, raw vegetables!

If you are not accustomed to making your own salad, use the following recipe to begin.

2 leaves of red leaf lettuce	1 carrot, sliced
2 leaves of green leaf lettuce	1 cucumber, sliced
1 cup spinach leaves	1 squash, sliced
1/2 cup dandelion leaves	1 tomato, diced

Wash and drain all vegetables. Run the carrot, cucumber, and squash through your salad shooter or slice them as thinly as possible. Dice the tomato. Break the lettuce, spinach, and dandelion into bite size pieces. Toss all ingredients into a large bowl. Makes four generous servings.

Fruit Salad

Mix together whatever fruits you have on hand. Some suggestions are apples, grapes, bananas, pineapple, plums, peaches, and pears. Sprinkle with fresh coconut and/or add lecithin granules. These fruits are delicious without a salad dressing, but if you must add something, try a little plain yogurt. The best plan is to eat fruit alone and on an empty stomach. Almost all fruit will digest within half an hour. Bananas digest within 45 minutes. If you eat fruit with a meal, it may ferment and cause bloating. Eat a celery stalk or lettuce leaves with your fruit to reduce this risk. These highly alkaline vegetables neutralize the acid in the stomach and help prevent bloating.

If you have never made a fruit salad, you might begin by trying the following recipe.

3 apples, diced	1 cup whole seedless grapes
3 peaches, diced	2 bananas, sliced
1 fresh pineapple, diced	6 ounces pineapple juice

Cut the pineapple shell, remove and dice the pineapple. Several ounces of juice will be expelled from the pineapple. Set the juice aside in a medium size bowl.

Peel and dice the apples. Slice the bananas. Place the apples and bananas in the pineapple juice. Be sure the fruit is covered with juice about ten seconds, then remove the fruit and place in a colander to drain. This keeps the apples and bananas from turning dark. Lemon juice has the same effect, but does not have the sweetness of pineapple juice. While the apples and bananas are draining, peel and dice the peaches. Now you are ready to toss together the apples, peaches, bananas, pineapple, and grapes. Sprinkle with a few lecithin granules if desired. Makes four generous servings.

Chapter 5

GRAINS AND
LEGUMES

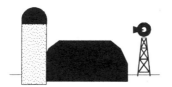

A land of wheat and barley....Deuteronomy 8:8

Grains and Legumes

Research has shown that dried beans and peas lower blood fats and decrease hardening of the arteries. Legumes combine very well with whole grains to make a complete protein. Both legumes and grains contain amino acids. Most grains contain a deficient amount of lysine but ample amounts of methionine. On the other hand, legumes are somewhat deficient in methionine but have an abundant amount of lysine.

If you eat grains or legumes alone, you will get some protein but not a complete protein. Grains and legumes combined provide an ideal balance of the essential amino acids. This makes the protein more easily assimilated by the body.

Season your legumes with onions, garlic, leeks, oregano, basil, tarragon, parsley, or any other herb or spice you might like. Add liquid aminos. Not only do these seasonings add flavor; they have medicinal value. Do not use fat or meat for seasoning; herbs are delicious and much more healthful. Use the legume recipes in this book to get started; then experiment with your own tastes and ideas.

Remember to eat whole grains with your legumes. Some suggestions are brown rice, amaranth, quinoa, millet, barley, and corn. Purchase whole grains - not processed - and follow the directions on the package. Use herbs to season your grains - garlic is excellent! You might also experiment with small amounts of tarragon, oregano, basil, and thyme.

Grain Experiment: Measure one cup of an uncooked grain of your choice. Follow cooking directions on the package. Add one teaspoon of one dried herb. The next time you prepare that grain, use a different herb. Enjoy several tasty and healthful combinations.

Navy Beans
(may also be used for blackeye peas)

1 cup Navy beans   1 large onion or leek
1 quart water   2 stalks celery
1 teaspoon salt   2 teaspoons liquid aminos

Wash the beans and soak them at least three hours or overnight. Drain and rinse again. Place them in a quart of boiling water. Add salt and all other ingredients. Bring to a boil and regulate heat. Partly cover, leaving an opening for steam to escape so the beans will not boil over. Stir every half hour and add more water if needed. Navy beans will need to cook about two hours or until well done.

Lentil Roast

1 cup red lentils (brown lentils if desired)
2 1/4 cups water
1 large onion, chopped 1 Tablespoon parsley flakes
2 stalks celery, chopped 1/8 teaspoon sweet basil
1 egg, slightly beaten   1/4 cup liquid aminos
1 cup grated mozzarella cheese or rice cheese

Rinse lentils and simmer in water and liquid aminos (covered) 25 minutes or until soft. Do not drain. Place onion, celery, egg, and basil in a large bowl and mix thoroughly. Add the lentils and mix again. Pour into a 9" square baking dish. Cover with grated cheese and sprinkle with parsley. Bake 25 minutes at 350 degrees.

Quinoa

Add 1 cup quinoa to 2 cups water. Bring to a boil; then simmer 15 minutes or until all water is absorbed. Season with 1/2 teaspoon salt and 1 teaspoon garlic powder. Serve with a dish of legumes.

Lentil/Rice Casserole

3/4 cup lentils
1/2 cup brown rice
1 medium onion
1 garlic clove
1 stalk celery
1/2 cup grated cheese
parsley

1 teaspoon salt
1/2 teaspoon basil
1/2 teaspoon oregano
1/4 teaspoon thyme
3 cups water
1 Tablespoon liquid aminos

Wash lentils and rice. Place in a casserole dish with 3 cups water. Chop the onion, celery, and garlic, and add them to the mixture. Now add the liquid aminos, salt, basil, oregano, and thyme. Cover and bake 1 1/2 hours at 300 degrees.

Remove from the oven and stir in the grated cheese. The casserole should be nearly done. If it appears a little dry, add some hot water (1/4 to 1/2 cup). Cover and return to the oven. Bake another 30 minutes. Before serving, sprinkle with parsley.

Just Lentils

Unlike many other legumes, lentils cook within half an hour. It is not necessary to soak them before cooking. Simply wash the lentils and put about 2 1/2 cups water to 1 cup lentils, 1 teaspoon salt, and a chopped onion or leek. If you are in a hurry and do not have time to prepare the onion or leek, substitute a generous spray (about two teaspoons) liquid aminos. Although hasty, it is tasty!

Amaranth

Add one cup of Amaranth to 3 cups boiling water. Season with 1/2 teaspoon salt and 1/2 teaspoon thyme. Bring to a second boil, reduce heat and simmer 30 minutes. Grains will absorb water and bind together. Serve with legumes.

Red Beans and Rice

5 cups water
1 cup red beans (or black beans)
1 cup brown rice
1 stalk celery, chopped

1 teaspoon salt
1 teaspoon garlic
1/4 cup liquid aminos

Soak beans several hours or overnight. Drain and discard the soaking water. Bring four cups of water to a boil and add beans, celery, salt, garlic, and liquid aminos. Bring to another boil, reduce temperature to medium low, cover and cook 1 1/2 hours. Add the rice. If necessary, add one more cup of water. Again bring to a boil, reduce heat and simmer until done. It takes approximately 45 minutes.

Brown Rice

3 cups water
1 cup brown rice
1/4 cup liquid aminos

1 teaspoon salt
1 teaspoon oregano

Bring water to a boil. Add all ingredients. Bring to another boil, reduce heat, and simmer 45 minutes.

This is only one recipe for brown rice. There are so many ways to prepare it, you can serve it a different way every day for at least a week. Add it to casseroles and soups or simply use the above basic recipe and flavor with various herbs. In place of oregano, use tarragon, garlic, thyme, rosemary, or whatever you like.

Brown rice is high in B vitamins as well as vitamin C. Create your own recipes for it and eat it often.

See the soup section (page 48) for more legume and grain recipes.

Chapter 6

VALUABLE

VEGETABLES

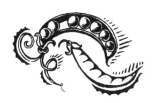

*And the Lord
God planted a
garden.....
Genesis 2:8*

Vegetables

You get the most nutritional value when you eat your vegetables raw. The fresher, the more nutritious. Raw foods are loaded with enzymes. Steamed vegetables possibly lose some of their enzymes, but not all. Although not as nutritious as raw vegetables, they still have a number of essential vitamins and minerals.

Most green and yellow vegetables (as well as some fruits) are excellent sources of beta carotene. Those containing significant amounts are asparagus, beets, broccoli, carrots, garlic, parsley, red peppers, spinach, sweet potatoes, yellow squash, and turnip greens. I specifically mentioned beta carotene because it is an excellent way to get Vitamin A, a powerful antioxidant.

One advantage of eating raw vegetables is that they raise the alkaline level in the body. If you are accustomed to eating junk foods, fast foods, white bread, sugar, and a high meat diet, chances are your body is acid. Viruses and diseases thrive in an acid environment. The best way to rid your body of excess acid is to counteract it with alkaline.

Celery is one of the best sources of alkaline foods. A stalk of celery has been known to ease the pain and discomfort of heartburn and to stop bloating. Other vegetables that serve this same role are cucumbers, red or green bell peppers, and lettuce leaves. Incidentally, green or red leaf lettuce has more nutritional value than iceberg lettuce.

Those suffering from candidiasis may experience discomfort as a result of eating fruit. This can be eliminated by eating celery stalks and/or lettuce leaves along with the fruit. Eat your fruit on an empty stomach and wait half an hour before eating anything else. Anyone suffering from candidiasis should consult a health practitioner before eating fruit.

Steamed Vegetables

If you have an automatic steamer, use it. Twenty minutes of steaming time gives most vegetables a good texture with the right amount of crunch. Some vegetables such as squash, okra, cauliflower, and broccoli should not be steamed longer than ten minutes. Use this recipe as a guide; then steam according to your taste.

2 large carrots	1 cauliflower
1 medium red skinned potato	1 bunch broccoli
1 cup green beans	15-20 pods okra

Wash and scrub all vegetables thoroughly. Slice the carrots and potato. Break the green beans into 1-inch pieces. Cut the cauliflower and broccoli into 1-inch florets or the size you desire. The okra will need very little preparation beyond cleaning.

Fill your steamer with the correct amount of water. Place the carrots, potato, and beans in the steam basket, cover and set the timer for 10 minutes. Now add the okra, broccoli, and cauliflower. Steam another 10 minutes.

Caution: Be careful when you remove your steamer lid to add the remaining vegetables. Use heavy cloths and keep your fingers away from the steam! Steam burns.

If you do not have a steamer, perhaps you can make one. Use a deep boiler with a lid and a colander that will fit inside it without touching bottom. Put one cup of water in the boiler, bring it to a boil, place vegetables in colander inside boiler, cover and steam. Experiment until you find the right temperature on your stove for steaming. It is usually medium-low.

Although I emphasize the value of raw and steamed vegetables, I have written several recipes for cooked vegetables, including stews. While it is true that cooking kills enzymes, home cooked vegetables still have some nutritional value. Adding raw vegetables to your meal will supply your body with enzymes to digest the cooked foods.

Vegetable Stew # 1

5 to 6 cups of water or vegetable broth
1 cup blackeye peas
1 cup fresh green beans
2 medium red skinned potatoes
1 cup baby lima beans
4 large carrots
2 stalks celery
1 medium onion
1 teaspoon garlic
2 teaspoons salt
2 Tablespoons liquid aminos

Use dried blackeye peas and baby limas is you can. Soak them overnight. Whether dried, fresh, or frozen, cook them together until they are almost done. While they are cooking, slice the onion, celery, carrots, and potatoes. Now snap the green beans.

You may add the onion, celery, garlic, salt, and liquid aminos to the peas and beans at any time. When they are almost done, add the potatoes and carrots. Boil rapidly ten minutes; then add the green beans. The green beans require less cooking time, so they should be added last.

You might need to add water as you add the other vegetables to the peas and beans. Use hot water; cold can slow the cooking process.

Vegetable Stew # 2

2 cups water or vegetable broth
2 medium red skinned potatoes
1 medium onion
2 stalks celery
2 Tablespoons arrowroot powder

4 large carrots
1/2 cup sweet peas
1 teaspoon salt
1 cup broccoli

Bring the water to a boil, add salt, and boil the carrots and potatoes 15 minutes. While they are boiling, slice or dice the onion and celery and drop them into the pot. When the water starts boiling again, add the peas. Let the stew come to another boil and add the broccoli and arrowroot powder. Boil five minutes. Remove from heat. Cover and seal in the heat as much as possible for 10 minutes before serving.

Vegetable Stew # 3

1 cup cauliflower, chopped
1 cup sweet peas
1 cup corn
1 cup water

1 leek
1 teaspoon garlic
1 teaspoon salt
1 Tablespoon liquid aminos

Bring all ingredients to a boil and simmer five to six minutes. Do not overcook.

Cooking A Vegetable Alone

Perhaps you would like to cook only one vegetable at the time, for instance a pot of corn or a pot sweet peas. Actual stovetop cooking time for these is 5-7 minutes. Most other vegetables will cook within 20 minutes.

Brown Rice & Sweet Peas

1 cup brown rice	1 teaspoon salt
3 cups water	1 leek, sliced
1 cup sweet peas	1 Tablespoon liquid aminos

Bring water to a boil. Add salt, rice, and leek. Simmer partly covered 40 minutes. Add peas and liquid aminos; bring to a boil again, and cook another 5 minutes.

Potatoes

Although all potatoes are nutritional, I prefer the red skinned potato. Whatever your preference, please don't peel your potatoes! When potatoes are peeled, the alkaline part is cut away and the potato is left lifeless and acid.

Baked Potatoes: A medium size potato will bake in 45 minutes. You can half it and season it with chives and liquid aminos. Add salt and pepper if desired. Never eat the potato without the skin.

Mashed potatoes: Scrub, cut, and boil the potatoes 20 minutes or until done. Pour off excess water, leaving enough to scarcely cover the potatoes. Beat with a mixer (skins and all) and season with a little salt and a lot of chives. Garnish with parsley if desired.

Baked Yellow Squash

Scrub the squash but do not peel. For medium squash, bake at 350 degrees for 20 minutes. To serve, cut in half like a baked potato. Season with salt and pepper if desired. Liquid aminos, thyme, oregano, chives, and parsley make excellent seasonings.

Baked Sweet Potatoes

Baked sweet potatoes are delicious. It takes about an hour to bake the large ones. Just slice them in half and eat them plain or sprinkle with ginger or cinnamon. If you must use butter, use only a small amount.

Sweet Potato Casserole

2 large or 4 medium sweet potatoes, baked and mashed

2 eggs, beaten	1 teaspoon vanilla
1/3 cup honey	1/3 cup milk
1/2 cup butter	1 cup fresh coconut
	(optional, but very tasty)

Topping for Sweet Potato Casserole

1/4 cup lecithin granules

1/3 cup honey	3/4 cups wheat flour
1 cup chopped nuts	2 Tablespoons melted butter

Mix ingredients for sweet potato casserole and place in a 9" square baking dish. Then mix topping. Topping should be crumbly. Spread evenly over casserole. Bake at 350 degrees for 25 minutes. Six to eight servings.

Apple-Yam Delight

4 medium baked yams (or any variety of sweet potatoes)

5 or 6 medium apples	2 Tablespoons lecithin
1/2 cup honey	cinnamon

Peel and slice the baked yams. Place in a 9" square baking dish. Peel and slice apples. Place them over the yams. Now pour the honey over the apples and yams. Sprinkle lecithin and cinnamon on top. Bake 25 minutes at 325 degrees. Six to eight servings.

Chapter 7

SAVORY

SOUP

*Then Jacob gave Esau
bread and pottage of
lentils.....Genesis 25:34*

Soup

Soup is delicious anytime and especially in cold or rainy weather. There is no limit to what you can put in soup. I seldom ever make it the same way twice; I simply use what I have on hand. Use these recipes as guidelines to create your own.

Eat whole grain crackers with your soup. Once you begin to enjoy the taste and texture of whole grain, you will never again want the common white flour crackers that line the shelves of the average grocery store.

You can save toward your next pot of vegetable soup as you prepare your daily vegetables. Save the parts that you would normally discard, such as celery roots, carrot ends, etc. Wash everything thoroughly and boil 20 to 30 minutes. Save the broth and discard the vegetable pieces. Use the nutrient rich broth as opposed to plain water for making soups and stews.

Remember to check and stir your soup at ten to fifteen minute intervals to avoid sticking and scorching. Also, keep plenty of hot water on hand to add to your soup should it become too thick or dry.

For variety, use a dry soup mixture with organic natural ingredients from a health food store. There are several flavors - beef, chicken and vegetable flavors are excellent. You can add these to your homemade soups and stews or simply add them to hot water and enjoy a flavorful soup!

The following recipe for lentil soup is one on my favorites. When I make lentil soup, I think of the Genesis account of Esau selling his birthright to Jacob for bread and a pottage of lentils. I wouldn't go so far as to say that lentil soup is worth a birthright, but it is a complete protein!

Lentil Soup

5 cups water	1/4 cup millet
1 cup dried lentils	1/4 cup quinoa
1 medium onion, diced	1/4 cup sunflower seeds
1 leek, diced	1/8 cup flax seeds
1 stalk celery, diced	2 Tablespoons sesame seeds
1/4 cup liquid aminos	1 Tablespoon parsley

Pour water into a large pot and bring to a boil. Add all ingredients. Bring to a boil again, cover and cook slowly 45 minutes. Stir occasionally. Cook until completely done. Add hot water if needed. Serve with whole grain crackers. Makes seven or eight generous servings.

Split Pea Soup

3 cups water	2 stalks celery
1 cup dried split peas	1 teaspoon salt
1 medium onion	1 Tablespoon liquid aminos
1 garlic clove or 1 teaspoon garlic	

Pour water into a large pot and bring to a boil. Add all ingredients. Bring to a second boil, reduce heat, cover and simmer 40 - 45 minutes. Stir occasionally. The peas should be very soft. It they are not, cook a little longer. Split peas are one of the few dried vegetables that you do not need to soak before cooking. Makes four generous servings.

Navy Bean Soup

Cook Navy Beans according to the recipe on page 38 with the following changes. Use two large onions. Blend onions and celery in a small amount of water before cooking. When beans are completely done, blend 2 tablespoons arrowroot powder in a small amount of water and add to beans. Stir and simmer another five minutes.

Barley-Bean Soup

5 cups water	1 teaspoon salt
1 cup dried beans (mixed)	1/2 cup uncooked barley
1 leek or onion, chopped	2 Tablespoons liquid aminos
2 stalks celery, chopped	1/2 teaspoon parsley

Mix your own beans or use a good, natural bean mix. Soak overnight. Drain and discard soaking water. Bring the water to a boil and add the salt and beans. Prepare the celery and onion and add them along with the liquid aminos. Boil until all the beans are done. This may take 1 1/2 to 2 hours. Be sure to check each kind of bean, as some cook quicker than others. Add more water if necessary. When the beans are done, add the barley and let the soup boil another 20 minutes. Then turn the burner off, cover, and seal in the heat another 10 minutes. Stir in parsley before serving.

This dish is a complete protein. You can be creative with this basic recipe. For instance, if you don't have barley on hand, use the same amount of millet, quinoa, or another grain. As for the beans, you can use any combination.

A Word About Taste and Texture

If you have a problem with the texture of diced onion, celery, leeks, or garlic, there's an easy way out. Simply cut them into large chunks and place them in the blender with a small amount of water. You can blend or liquefy them. The taste and nutritional value are there without the texture. As you begin to eat more foods seasoned with herbs and spices, you will actually *like* the texture of these things.

Potato Soup

1 quart water
8 medium potatoes
1 carrot
1/4 teaspoon basil

1 medium onion
1 Tablespoon liquid aminos
1 teaspoon salt
1 Tablespoon chives

Pour the water into a 3-quart saucepan. Wash the potatoes, leave the peelings on, and grate two of the potatoes and the carrot to add thickness to the soup. Dice the remaining six potatoes. Place all ingredients in a quart of boiling water. Simmer partly covered until the potatoes are well done. It will take approximately 40 minutes. Makes four generous servings.

Cream of Carrot Soup

3 cups water
1 cup carrot pulp from juicing carrots
1 teaspoon salt
1 stalk celery, sliced
1 medium onion, sliced
1/2 teaspoon oregano
1 teaspoon chives
1 Tablespoon liquid aminos
1 Tablespoon arrowroot powder

Bring water to a boil. Add all ingredients and simmer 20 minutes, stirring frequently. Makes a quick, delicious meal for two people.

You may prefer to use sliced carrots as opposed to carrot pulp. Two or three carrots should be sufficient. Just simmer them about 20 minutes; there is no need to stir.

Chili

1/2 pound dry pinto or kidney beans
6 or 7 medium fresh tomatoes, chopped
1 pound ground turkey
2 medium onions, coarsely chopped
2 cloves garlic, crushed or chopped
2 Tablespoons chili peppers, chopped
1 teaspoon pepper
1 teaspoon cumin
Salt to taste

Soak dry beans overnight in two cups of water. Drain and wash thoroughly. Place in a 2-quart saucepan with two more cups of water and cook until done. Drain well. Cut tomatoes small enough to go into blender with a small amount of water (not more than 1/4 cup) and puree. Brown the turkey slowly in a skillet. Place beans, pureed tomatoes, turkey, and all other ingredients in crockpot and simmer 10 to 12 hours. Serves four.

If stovetop cooking is desired, place all ingredients in a large pot and simmer approximately three hours. Check frequently and add a little water if it tends to run dry.

NOTE: Be sure to read the ingredients on the package of turkey you buy. It should contain 100% ground turkey - no additives or preservatives.

Option: If you are one who insists that chili must be cooked with beef, not turkey, try to buy your beef from a farmer who raises cattle the natural way - no hormones or antibiotics. Although difficult, it is still possible to find this kind of beef in some areas. Question the butcher who cuts and wraps it. Insist that your beef not be processed with gamma ray.

Cream of Chickpea Soup

1 1/2 cups dried chickpeas (garbanzo beans)
1 cup onion, chopped   1 teaspoon salt
1 clove garlic, minced   1 celery stalk, chopped
6 cups water   1/4 cup chopped parsley

Place peas in a bowl with four cups of water. Refrigerate and soak overnight. Drain and wash thoroughly. Place all ingredients except parsley in six cups of water, bring to a boil, reduce heat, cover, and simmer for three hours. When peas are tender, strain and <u>save the broth</u>. As soon as peas are cool enough, pour into blender with just enough water to puree. Combine pureed peas with broth you strained, add parsley, and reheat. Serve hot.

This makes a thick, creamy soup. It is excellent for a "soup and salad" meal. It may also be used as a thickener for pot pies, stews, etc. Freeze leftovers and use later.

More About Soup

You don't really need a recipe for soup. As you work more with whole foods, you will soon know the cooking time for each vegetable and will be able to make quite a variety of soups.

When you have vegetables left over from a meal, consider making these into a soup for the next day. Most vegetables mix together quite well. Just throw them in the pot with water or broth, season them with your favorite herbs, and call the dish your "own original vegetable soup."

Chapter 8

PASTA HAS

IT'S PLACE

Pasta
and the truth about tomatoes

When we think "pasta," we usually think spaghetti, lasagna, or some kind of noodles cooked with tomato sauce. I never recommend that cooked tomatoes be eaten more than once a week. Although raw tomatoes contain citric acid, they are an alkaline forming food, whereas cooked tomatoes are extremely acid forming.

If you possibly can, you should make your own sauce from fresh tomatoes. Although you will cook the tomatoes, the sauce will be much more nutritional than a ready prepared sauce. Never use sauce from a can or canned tomatoes to make your sauce. If you feel that you simply cannot make your own sauce, shop carefully for a healthful sauce in a jar. Avoid sauces containing sugar and high fructose syrup. It may be necessary to purchase your sauce from a health food store.

For our first pasta, let's begin with a recipe that does not include tomatoes. It's a delicious non-dairy dish of macaroni and cheese!

Macaroni & Cheese

1 8-oz. package Quinoa noodles
1 8-oz. package rice cheese, soy cheese, or dairy cheese
        with no food coloring or dyes
1 teaspoon salt
1 Tablespoon liquid aminos

Cook the noodles according to directions on the package. Add salt. Drain most of the water out. Leave a very small amount to help stir in the cheese. Add liquid aminos and heat again on low if necessary. Four to six servings.

Homemade Spaghetti Sauce

10 medium or large fresh tomatoes
1/4 cup water
2 Tablespoons olive oil
1 garlic clove or one teaspoon garlic
1 large onion
1 stalk celery
1 teaspoon salt
1/4 cup fresh parsley
1/8 cup basil
1/8 cup oregano
1/8 cup liquid aminos

Puree the tomatoes, onion, and celery in the blender. This mixture will puree easier if you add the 1/4 cup water. Now place in a saucepan and add the other ingredients. Cover and simmer over low heat approximately one hour, stirring occasionally.

If you prefer cooking this in your crockpot, don't add the 1/4 cup water. The crockpot tends to hold the liquids in more. Use the lowest setting and let it cook about eight hours.

This sauce may be used for lasagna, spaghetti, or pizza.

Another word of caution: Most children like spaghetti and other forms of cooked tomatoes. It is up to you to limit their intake of these items. When you do allow them to eat these foods, insist that they eat a large vegetable salad along with their spaghetti, lasagna, pizza, etc. This is also a good rule for you to follow. You don't want to overload the body with acid. Remember, germs thrive in an acid environment. The raw salad will fight germs by raising the body's alkaline level and by providing enzymes vital to digestion.

Pizza Crust
(may also be used for pot pies)

1 1/2 teaspoons yeast
1/2 cup warm water
1 teaspoon baking soda
1/4 teaspoon salt
1 Tablespoon olive oil
1 Tablespoon honey
1 1/4 cups flour, sifted
Approximately 1/2 cup extra flour

Dissolve the yeast in the warm water. Add the baking soda, salt, oil, honey, and flour. Flour a kneading board with the extra flour. Roll dough on floured board to desired thickness. This makes enough to cover a large cookie sheet or two 9" pans.

Pizza

Pizza crust (see preceding recipe)
Spaghetti sauce on page 57
        (or buy a 16-ounce jar)
Parsley
1 teaspoon garlic powder
8 ounces grated all natural mozzarella cheese

Spoon spaghetti sauce generously over crust. Sprinkle a little garlic and parsley over the sauce; then cover generously with cheese. Bake 20 minutes at 300 degrees.

Tip: Pizza crusts may be baked and frozen for later use. Remove them from the freezer and proceed with the above pizza recipe.

Spaghetti And Meatballs

Sauce
One 32 oz. jar of natural spaghetti sauce
(or make your own)

Meatballs

1 lb. ground turkey or beef
Salt and pepper (sprinkled as desired)
1 teaspoon or 1 clove garlic
1 large onion
1 egg (beaten)
2 Tablespoons parsley
1 teaspoon oregano
1/2 teaspoon basil
1 Tablespoon liquid aminos
1 cup flour

Puree onion and garlic. Salt and pepper the meat. Add all other ingredients except the flour. Mix thoroughly with a spoon. Now add the flour and stir it into the mixture.

Butter a large skillet. Form the mixture into meatballs and place in the skillet. Cover and simmer on low heat until done. It takes about 20 minutes. Turn once after 10 minutes. Pour the spaghetti sauce over the meatballs and simmer approximately another half hour.

Pasta (noodles)

One 8-oz. package of Jerusalem Artichoke noodles or
        Tomato & Basil noodles
Follow cooking directions on package. Salt to taste.

Add meat and sauce to pasta and serve. Makes six to eight generous servings.

Spaghetti Sauce With Meat

1 32-ounce jar of spaghetti sauce (or make your own)
1 lb. ground turkey or beef
salt and pepper (sprinkled as desired)
1 teaspoon or 1 clove garlic, minced   1/2 teaspoon basil
1 large onion, chopped   2 Tablespoons parsley
1 Tablespoon liquid aminos   1 teaspoon oregano

Salt and pepper meat. Simmer over low heat until brown.
Drain the fat off. Place in covered skillet or saucepan with
all other ingredients and simmer 30 minutes. Excellent for
spaghetti pie.

Spaghetti Pie

Pie Crust: Cooked spaghetti noodles (page 59)
Pie Filling: Spaghetti sauce with meat (above)
Pie Topping: 8 ounces grated mozzarella cheese

Put your pie together in a 9"x13" baking dish and bake 25
minutes at 300 degrees. Makes 6 - 8 generous servings.

Lasagna

1 8-oz. pkg. of Lasagna noodles made from whole grains
Use the above recipe for Spaghetti sauce with meat
16 ounces grated mozzarella cheese

Cook the noodles following the directions on the package.
Salt to taste. Drain. Place one layer of cooked noodles in a
9"x13" baking dish. Place a layer of sauce and then a layer
of cheese. Repeat once or twice more. Bake 30 minutes at
350 degrees. Makes six to eight servings.

Chapter 9

EAT

MEAT?

Every moving thing that liveth shall be meat for you; even as the green herb have I given you all things. Genesis 9:3

Meat

Unlike many nutritionists, I have no problem with eating meat. However, I will acknowledge the fact that the body has more difficulty digesting meat than it does fruits, vegetables, nuts, and seeds. Ideally, meat should not be eaten every day. Three times each week is sufficient. There are many excellent sources of protein aside from meat. For someone who has a serious digestive problem or an autoimmune disorder, it is wise to eat very little meat.

I have heard it said that God gave Adam and Eve plants and herbs to eat. That is correct. However, God permitted Noah and his family to eat meat after the flood. Meat was simply added to the diet; it was never meant to take the place of plants and herbs.

The eighteenth chapter of Genesis relates the account of Abraham's servant preparing a calf along with milk and butter for a special occasion. Abraham was entertaining angels who brought to him the promise of a son in his old age.

Most of us are familiar with the story of the prodigal son in Luke 15. The glad father rejoiced when he saw his son coming home. That called for a real celebration, so he killed the fatted calf.

It is recorded in Luke 24 that when Jesus was with His disciples after the resurrection, He ate a piece of broiled fish and a honeycomb. Incidentally, a little honey is delicious with fish!

Perhaps we should eat meat only on special occasions. Surely there would be health benefits in doing this.

Turkey Patties
(also works well with beef or ostrich patties)

1 pound ground all natural turkey
Salt and pepper sprinkled over the meat
1/2 teaspoon garlic powder or 1 garlic clove, sliced
1/2 teaspoon oregano
1/4 teaspoon basil
1 Tablespoon tarragon
1 medium onion, diced
2 Tablespoons liquid aminos
1 cup flour

Mix all ingredients together. Use the flour for forming patties and holding them together. Make the patties any size you like. Place them in a large buttered skillet. Cover and simmer until both sides are golden brown. They will need to cook approximately 15 to 20 minutes on each side.

Serve homemade biscuits with your patties. A patty inside a biscuit makes a delicious sandwich.

Baked Turkey
(season with salt and sage)

Shop for a natural turkey - not injected. Clean well, season with salt and sage, place in a large covered baking dish, cover and bake slowly. Turkey is delicious when baked at 200 degrees overnight. If this is not possible, bake at 325 degrees, allowing 30 minutes baking time per pound. Let cool and remove from bone. Place in freezer bags and freeze for future use.

Baked turkey may be served in slices with a meal, used for sandwiches, or used in casseroles. Use the Chicken/Rice recipe on page 66 to make Turkey/Rice Casserole.

Chicken

If you can possibly buy your chickens from a farmer who cares for and feeds his chickens properly, please do so. If not, read the label carefully. Search for a statement about the chicken being "all natural." Look for any indication that the chicken has been given hormones or injected with any substance "to preserve freshness." It is wise to avoid injected chickens.

Chicken can be prepared a number of ways. You can bake a chicken, pull the meat off the bones, and freeze for later use. Use it to make sandwiches, chicken salad, or to supplement a meal.

Chicken Broth

Baking a chicken produces fat drippings. Add one cup of water to each cup of fat to make a broth. If you boil the chicken, the water you boil it in becomes broth. Chicken broth may be used to make dressing, dumplings, soup, and other delicious chicken dishes. If you limit your use of chicken broth or turkey broth to one time per week, you should not worry about the fat. You need some fat in your diet, and this is one of the better ways to get it. However, if you prefer not to eat the fat, simply skim it off the broth.

Oregano Chicken

1 whole chicken	Oregano
Salt	1/2 to 1 cup water

Wash the chicken thoroughly and sprinkle with salt and oregano. Be generous with the oregano. Bake in a covered dish 1 1/2 hours at 350 degrees or cook on low setting in the crockpot eight to ten hours. Add water - no more than one cup - to prevent dryness.

Chicken and Dumplings

1 cooked chicken removed from bone
4-5 cups liquid made of chicken broth and water

1 cup warm buttermilk (not hot)	2 cups flour
2 Tablespoons olive oil	1 teaspoon salt
1/2 teaspoons Xanthan gum	1 Tablespoon gluten
1 Tablespoon baking powder	Salt and pepper

Either boil or bake the chicken until completely done. Let cool and remove the meat from the bone. Add enough water to the chicken broth to make 4-5 cups liquid. Do not put the chicken in the broth until you have cooked the dumplings.

Pour the broth into a large pot and turn the burner on medium high. While the broth is heating, flour a kneading board to use for rolling your dumplings. If you do not have a kneading board, use a large cloth, the gummed side of aluminum foil, freezer paper, or wax paper. Now you are ready to make dumplings.

Warm the buttermilk on low heat and set aside. Sift and measure flour. Make a large crevice in the middle of the flour. Pour the baking powder, salt, gluten, and Xanthan gum into the crevice. Now pour the olive oil into the crevice. Stirring from the center, slowly add the warm buttermilk. Bring the flour a little at the time into the mixture. Continue stirring until the dough becomes thick and is coated with flour. Use excess flour for rolling.

Be sure the broth is boiling. Now place the dough on a floured board or cloth. Roll with floured rolling pin until very thin. Add additional flour as necessary. Cut in squares about 1 1/2 inches and drop into rapidly boiling broth. Stir frequently and boil seven minutes. Now add the chicken, salt and papper, stir again, remove from heat and cover. Let it remain covered ten minutes. Serves 6-8 people.

Chicken/Rice Casserole

1 whole baked chicken
1 cup chicken broth
1 stalk celery, chopped
1 teaspoon salt
4 carrots, sliced
2/3 cup sweet peas

1 cup brown rice
4 cups water
1 onion, chopped
1 teaspoon sage
2 Tablespoons liquid aminos

Pull baked chicken off the bone and remove all skin. Place it along with 1 cup broth, 4 cups water, and 1 cup rice in a large baking dish. Slice and place all vegetables around the chicken. Sprinkle the seasonings on the chicken and vegetables. You may use other vegetables such as cauliflower, broccoli, or whatever you have on hand. Bake covered at 350 degrees for 1 1/2 hours. Serves 4-6 people.

This may seem a long time to cook vegetables, but it takes this long for the rice to cook in the oven. If you prefer to not cook your vegetables this long, place only the chicken, broth, rice, salt, onion, celery, and sage in the dish and bake 45 minutes. Then add the remaining ingredients and bake another 45 minutes.

Chicken Pie

2 cups diced chicken
2 teaspoons salt
2 large carrots
2 medium potatoes
1/2 cup sweet peas

2 stalks celery, chopped
1 leek or onion, chopped
1 teaspoon garlic
2 Tablespoons liquid aminos
2 cups cream of chickpea soup
(see recipe on page 54)

Stir all ingredients together and place in a large baking dish. Make a crust and place on top. See page 58 for a yeast crust or page 72 for a regular pie crust. Bake at 325 degrees 45 minutes. Serves 4-6 people.

Chicken and Dressing

One baked chicken   2 boiled eggs
3 cups cornbread crumbs   1 Tablespoon oregano
1 onion   1 Tablespoon parsley
2 stalks celery   1/4 cup liquid aminos
3 cups chicken broth   1/2 teaspoon sage

Salt and bake the chicken. Let it cool and remove bone. If you plan to make gravy, dice 1/4 cup of the chicken and set aside.

Make the cornbread (page 29) and break it into crumbs. Dice the boiled eggs. You may either dice the onion and celery or blend them. Use a natural chicken broth - not canned - without preservatives or artificial ingredients.

Stir all ingredients together. Serve the chicken as a separate dish or mix it with the dressing. It's good both ways. Bake in a covered casserole dish 1 hour at 325 degrees. Serves 6-8.

Gravy

1 leek   1 cup chicken broth   1/4 cup diced chicken
3 Tablespoons arrowroot powder or 6 Tablespoons flour

Blend the leek, flour, and chicken broth. Simmer two to three minutes and stir in diced chicken. Continue stirring until the gravy reaches its desired thickness. If it becomes too thick, add a little water. Serve with dressing, mashed potatoes, or brown rice.

Beef

If you have access to hormone free beef, try the following recipes. Unless you have been advised to not eat beef for health reasons, it can safely be eaten once or twice each week. Trim as much of the fat as you can from your roasts, steaks, and stew beef, and cook your meat well done.

Roast With Vegetables

Roast (approx. 3 lbs.)   1 large onion (dice or blend)
1/2 cup water   6 carrots, sliced
2 Tablespoons liquid aminos   4 medium potatoes, sliced

Place roast in a large casserole dish with water, onion, liquid aminos, carrots, and potatoes. Salt and pepper the meat and vegetables. Cover the dish. If you do not have a covered casserole dish, use aluminum foil, making sure the gummed side (not the shiny side) is near the food. Bake 6 to 7 hours (or overnight) at 250 degrees. The roast will be so tender you will not need a knife to cut it.

Stew Beef

1 lb. lean beef stew, salted and peppered
3 cups water   1 large onion (dice or blend)

Place all ingredients in a 2-quart saucepan and bring to a boil. Reduce heat, cover and simmer 2 hours or until meat is tender. If you wish to add vegetables such as carrots and potatoes, do so after the meat is done, and cook an additional 20 to 30 minutes. For a thickener, blend 2 tablespoons arrowroot powder in 1/4 cup of water. Stir into the stew and cook two additional minutes. Serve over brown rice.

Fish

A meal of fresh fish is hard to beat. For a fish feast, allow 1/2 pound of fillets per person. Bake, broil, grill, or steam your fish. Here's my favorite way to cook fish.

Dip fish fillets in a mixture of lemon juice and liquid aminos. Place them on a broiling pan. Salt and pepper. Sprinkle with garlic. Broil at a high temperature. It takes about 20 minutes. Serve with your favorite legumes, rice, and salad. Steamed vegetables are also good with fish. Mary's Garlic Bread (page 31) tops it off!

Try a little honey with your fish. Jesus ate it that way so it has to be good! If you have any fish left over, make fish chowder.

Fish Chowder

1 quart vegetable broth or water
Leftover fish, one to two cups, cut or diced (all bones out)

1 potato, cubed or sliced	1 teaspoon garlic
1/2 cup sweet peas	2 tomatoes, diced
1 or 2 carrots, sliced	1 onion, chopped
Salt and pepper to taste	

Place all ingredients except fish in a large pot. Boil 30 minutes, add fish and boil another two to three minutes. Serve hot with whole grain crackers.

If you have a good vegetable broth on hand, use it to make your chowder. If you use water, add 1/4 cup liquid aminos. Chop a stalk of celery and a leek or an onion. Add these to enhance the flavor. Remember, you can blend all these things if you desire a "smooth" soup texture.

Chapter 10

DELICIOUS

DESSERTS

Dessert is a treat; don't overeat!

Desserts

Do you feel that you must have a dessert with every meal? As you rid your body of the foods that contain toxins, your tastes will change. You will become "addicted" to healthful foods. When you do eat desserts, don't eat those containing sugar or synthetic preservatives. Here are some tasty and healthful recipes.

Pineapple Cake

1/2 cup butter	2 cups whole wheat flour
2/3 cup honey	2 teaspoon baking soda
3 eggs separated	1/2 teaspoon salt
1 cup fresh diced pineapple	
1/2 cup pineapple juice or apple juice	

Cream butter and honey. Add egg yolks and beat until light. Stir in dry ingredients. Add juice and mix thoroughly. Fold in pineapple and beaten egg whites. Pour into buttered 9"x13" dish and bake 55 minutes at 350 degrees.

For a pineapple upside down cake: Extra pineapple (sliced) may be used to line the baking dish. Pour the cake mixture over it and bake. Let cool. Place a serving plate on top of the pan. Invert both, then lift off pan.

Frosting for Pineapple Cake

1/4 cup butter	1 teaspoon vanilla
1/2 c. honey or maple syrup	2 Tablespoons pineapple juice
1/2 cup soy milk powder or rice milk powder	
1 cup diced pineapple	

Cream together the butter, honey, vanilla, and juice. Stir in milk powder. Spread over cake. Garnish with diced pineapple.

Peach Cobbler

3/4 cup milk   3/4 cup flour
1/2 cup honey   1/2 cup butter
2 cups fresh sliced peaches

Mix milk, honey, flour, and butter. Pour into a deep baking dish. Place peaches on top. Bake at 350 degrees one hour.

Coconut Pie

1/2 cup honey   3 eggs
3 Tablespoons flour   1/2 cup butter
A pinch of salt   1 cup milk
2 cups fresh shredded coconut

Beat eggs. Add butter and honey and mix well. Mix in all dry ingredients and add milk. Beat on medium speed until all ingredients are thoroughly mixed. Now stir in coconut. Pour into a 9" unbaked pie shell and bake 45 minutes at 325 degrees.

Pie Crust

3/4 cup flour   1/4 teaspoon salt
1 teaspoon baking powder   1 Tablespoon olive oil
1/2 cup water

Mix with a spoon and knead well with fingers. Roll onto a well floured kneading board until very thin. Place in a 9" pie plate and shape dough around the edges. Use a fork for decorative design.

The pie crust may be pre-baked 10 minutes at 425 degrees or used as an unbaked pie crust.

Party Cake

3 whole eggs or 2 egg yolks + 2 whole eggs
(the two extra egg whites may be used for frosting)

1/2 cup butter	3/4 cup honey
3/4 cup buttermilk	1 1/2 teaspoon vanilla extract
2 c. unbleached white flour	1 teaspoon salt
1/2 cup whole wheat flour	2 teaspoons baking soda

Optional: 1 teaspoon almond extract

Beat egg whites until stiff and set aside. Beat egg yolks. Add butter, honey, and buttermilk. Mix well. Combine with dry ingredients and beat thoroughly on medium speed. Add vanilla (and almond if desired). Fold egg whites into mixture. Pour into a buttered 9"x13" pan and bake 40 minutes at 350 degrees. Let cool. Place a serving plate or board on top of the pan. Invert both, then lift off pan. Ice the cake and decorate it for a birthday or other occasion.

For cupcakes, pour into muffin pans and bake 20 minutes at 325 degrees. Makes approximately 12-15 muffins.

Icing

2 egg whites, beaten	1/8 teaspoon salt
1/2 cup honey	1 teaspoon vanilla extract
1/4 teaspoon cream of tarter	

Use a double boiler. After water is boiling well, place all ingredients except vanilla in the top of the double boiler and beat 7-10 minutes until frosting stands alone in peaks. Remove from heat, add vanilla, and continue beating one minute. Spread on cake immediately.

Tip: To ice the cake smoothly, dip the knife in hot water before spreading the icing.

Brownies

2 eggs	1/2 teaspoon salt
2/3 cup honey	1 teaspoon baking soda
1/2 cup melted butter	3/4 cup water
1 teaspoon vanilla	1/3 cup carob powder, sifted
1 banana, mashed	1 cup whole wheat flour
1/2 cup raisins	1 cup chopped walnuts

Beat eggs. Add butter, honey, vanilla, and banana. Beat again. Add the flour, carob, salt, soda, and water. Beat well. Stir in the raisins and walnuts. Pour into a buttered 13"x9" glass baking dish and bake 25 minutes at 350 degrees.

Pound Cake

2 cups unbleached white flour	1 cup butter
1 cup whole wheat pastry flour	1 1/2 cups honey
1 teaspoon baking soda	5 eggs, separated
1 cup milk	1 teaspoon vanilla

Beat egg whites until stiff and set aside. Melt butter and let cool. Add honey and egg yolks. Beat on low speed until thoroughly mixed. Sift dry ingredients and stir in. Add buttermilk and vanilla. Mix thoroughly. Fold egg whites into mixture. Place in a buttered tube or bundt pan and bake 1 hour and 10 minutes at 325 degrees. Remove from oven and let cool before slicing.

About Apples

As a rule, I do not recommend peeling apples, as the peelings contain many nutrients. However, I do peel apples for making applesauce and apple crisp which you will find on the following page. Should you prefer to not peel your apples, just blend them well for the applesauce and consider the peelings as a "crispy" part of the apple crisp.

Applesauce

3 or 4 apples, peeled and sliced   1 ounce water
1 Tablespoon lecithin granules (optional)

Dip the diced apples in pineapple juice or lemon juice. This will prevent discoloring of the apples. Place all ingredients in the blender and puree. The water helps start the puree process. Apples are naturally sweet. There is no need to add a sweetener. The lecithin gives the applesauce a distinct flavor. May be eaten uncooked; however, if you wish to cook your applesauce, simmer 5 minutes on low heat.

Apple Crisp

4 cups peeled, diced apples   1/2 cup honey
1 1/2 cup uncooked oatmeal   1/4 cup walnut pieces
1 cup milk   1/4 cup almond pieces
1/2 cup whole wheat flour   1/4 cup cashews
2 Tablespoons lecithin   1/4 teaspoon cinnamon

Place the apples in a buttered 9" square baking dish. Sprinkle cinnamon over them and set aside. Sift the flour. Add honey and milk to the flour and beat until well mixed. Stir in the oatmeal, lecithin, and nuts. Pour this mixture over the apples and cinnamon. Bake at 350 degrees 35 minutes.

Strawberry Pie

2 cups red grape juice   1 Tablespoon honey
2 pkgs unflavored gelatin   2 pints strawberries, sliced

Heat grape juice but do not boil. Melt gelatin in juice, add honey and stir. Let cool while preparing strawberries. Wash and slice strawberries and place in a pre-baked cooled 9" pie shell (see page 72). Pour cooled juice mixture over strawberries and refrigerate two hours or until firm.

Fruitcake

1 cup flour
1 teaspoon baking soda
1/2 teaspoon salt
1/2 cup butter
1/2 cup honey
2 eggs
2 Tablespoons apple juice
1 cup chopped walnuts
1 cup chopped pecans
1/4 teaspoon nutmeg

Unsulphured Dried fruits:
1 cup pineapple, chopped
1/2 cup apples
1/2 cup apricots, chopped
1/2 cup raisins
1/2 cup dates, chopped
* * * * *
1 teaspoon fresh lemon peel
1 teaspoon fresh orange peel

Melt butter and mix with eggs, honey, and apple juice. Add nutmeg, flour, soda, and salt. Grate the lemon peel and orange peel. Stir these in the mixture along with all fruits and nuts. Continue to stir until all ingredients are thoroughly mixed. Pour into a buttered tube pan or bundt pan and bake 1 1/2 hours at 300 degrees. If you prefer a loaf pan, this will fill two average size loaf pans.

Oatmeal Cookies

2 cups whole wheat flour
1 teaspoon baking soda
1 teaspoon salt
3 cups oatmeal (100% rolled oats)
2 eggs, beaten

1 cup butter
1 cup honey
1 teaspoon vanilla

1 cup raisins (optional)
1 cup walnuts or pecans

Cream butter, honey, vanilla, and eggs. Add dry ingredients and stir until thoroughly mixed. Add raisins and/or nuts if desired. Drop onto buttered cookie sheet allowing space between cookies. Bake 12 to 15 minutes at 350 degrees. Makes about four dozen cookies.

Old Fashioned Ice Cream

3 Tablespoons flour	1/2 cup chopped almonds
2 eggs	2 medium bananas, mashed
1 quart milk	2 Tablespoons lecithin granules
1 Tablespoon vanilla	1/2 cup honey
1/2 cup coconut	2 teaspoons Xanthan gum (optional)

Blend flour, eggs, milk, lecithin granules, and Xanthan gum. Place in a saucepan over medium heat and bring to a boil. Cook two to three minutes (until it begins to thicken) stirring constantly. Remove from heat and stir in the honey, almonds, bananas, coconut, and vanilla. Pour into a large bowl and let cool 30 minutes, then place in freezer. For best results, remove from freezer after two hours and blend. Repeat after another two hours. Repead blending makes a smoother texture.

Be creative with this recipe. If you do not care for bananas and coconut, use strawberries, blueberries, etc. Perhaps you would prefer walnuts instead of almonds.

My nephew is a diabetic. His mother (my sister-in-law) makes ice cream by this recipe, using 1/4 teaspoon stevia (no honey) to sweeten it. She tried this same recipe using an ice cream freezer. The ice cream is much smoother and creamier when made in a freezer.

Xanthan gum helps make the ice cream smooth and creamy. The same amount of slippery elm may be used in its place.

If you like chocolate ice cream, experiment with carob. Use two tablespoons carob powder and one additional tablespoon honey. Carob contains a balance of calcium and phosphorus. Carob does not contain caffeine and does not interfere with calcium absorption as chocolate does.

Freezer Ice Cream

1/2 cup cashews	4 peaches, peeled and chopped
2 eggs	2 medium bananas, mashed
1 quart rice milk	2 Tablespoons lecithin granules
1/3 cup honey	2 teaspoons Xanthan gum (optional)
1 Tablespoon vanilla extract	

Blend all ingredients. Pour the milk into the blender last. If there is not enough room for all of it, blend only half of it with the other ingredients. Pour the mixture into the ice cream freezer and stir the remainder of the milk into the mixture.

Be creative. Use whatever fruit and nuts you have on hand. If you make the ice cream without using fruit to help sweeten it, you might need to increase the honey to 1/2 cup and the lecithin granules to 3 or 4 Tablespoons.

Add sliced bananas for a banana split.

Follow the directions for your ice cream freezer using ice and rock salt. Freezing time is approximately 30 minutes for most ice cream freezers.

Try garnishing your ice cream with bran flakes or raw nuts. It's delicious!

Strawberry Shortcake

Make cupcakes using the party cake recipe on page 73. Serve ice cream over a cupcake. Cover with fresh strawberries. If the strawberries are large, cut or dice them.

For variety, try peaches, bananas, or blueberries with your cake and ice cream.

Yogurt Ice Cream

2 cups plain yogurt   2 Tablespoons lecithin granules
2 eggs   1 cup honey
1 quart milk   2 Tablespoons vanilla
2 teaspoons Xanthan gum (optional)

Blend all ingredients. Pour the milk into the blender last. If there is not enough room for all of it, blend only half of it with the other ingredients. Pour the mixture into the ice cream freezer and stir the remainder of the milk into the mixture.

Ice cream maker method: Place into ice cream freezer and churn as you would any ice cream.

Freezer method: Blend and place in freezer. For best results, remove from freezer after two hours and blend again. For a smoother texture, repeat after another two hours.

Strawberry Yogurt

1 package unflavored gelatin   1/2 cup honey
1 ounce boiling water   1 cup milk
2 cups plain yogurt   2 cups strawberries
2 eggs   1 Tablespoon vanilla
1 teaspoon Xanthan gum

Pour boiling water over gelatin and stir until completely dissolved. Place dissolved gelatin, yogurt, eggs, honey, milk, and vanilla in blender and blend well. Add strawberries and blend again. Follow freezing instructions for yogurt ice cream (above).

Fruit Pies

Bake your favorite fruit pie (apple, peach, pear) using this recipe.

6 cups sliced fresh fruit	1/2 cup honey
2 Tablespoons butter	1/2 cup milk
1/4 cup flour	1/4 teaspoon cinnamon
2 pie crusts (page 72)	

Place uncooked pie crust in a 9-inch buttered pie pan. Place fruit evenly. Mix together butter, flour, honey, cinnamon, and milk. Pour over fruit and place second pie crust on top. Bake 30 to 35 minutes at 425 degrees.

Trail Mix

Excellent for parties or just a snack. Use the following ingredients. Add to them or change them to suit your own taste. Just be sure to use raw nuts and unsulphured fruits.

pine nuts	almonds
cashew nuts	raisins
sunflower seeds	dried bananas
pumpkin seeds	dried apricots

You may use any amount you wish; there is no set rule. If you insist on measuring everything, try 1/2 cup of each and stir until thoroughly mixed. This amount would be good for a party snack. If making a snack for a small family to eat at home, you would need to use considerably less, perhaps 1/8 cup of each.

Jello

4 envelopes unflavored gelatin   1 cup cold fruit juice
3 cups fruit juice, heated to boiling   1/2 cup dried apricots
1/4 cup dried raisins   1/4 cup dates
1/2 cup dried pineapple (chop if bought in rings)
1/4 cup sesame seeds or flax seeds (optional)

Use 1 1/2 cups of dried fruit. If there is a kind you do not have on hand or prefer not to use, substitute what you want.

Stir gelatin into hot juice until gelatin is dissolved. Stir in the cold juice and the dried fruits and seeds. Pour into a 13"x9" dish and chill until firm. It takes about two hours. Cut into 1-inch squares and serve. Makes enough for a large family.

Carrot Cake

2 eggs   1 teaspoon baking soda
1/2 cup butter   1/4 teaspoon salt
1 cup honey   1 teaspoon cinnamon
1/3 cup buttermilk   1 3/4 cups flour
1 cup grated carrots   1 cup walnuts, chopped

Mix together the eggs, butter, honey. In another bowl, sift the flour and add salt, cinnamon, and baking soda. Add the eggs, butter, and honey to the dry ingredients. Now add the buttermilk and mix thoroughly. Stir in carrots and walnuts. Pour into a buttered 9"x13" baking dish. Bake 30 to 35 minutes at 350 degrees.

Cream Cheese Icing

8 ounces cream cheese, softened
1 teaspoon vanilla   1/4 cup honey

Mix all ingredients until smooth. Spread over carrot cake.

Millet Balls

1 cup cooked millet
1/2 cup chopped walnuts
1/2 cup chopped almonds
1/2 cup chopped cashews
1/2 cup raisins
1/2 cup chopped dried apricots
1/2 cup chopped dried apples
2 Tablespoons water
2 Tablespoons pure maple syrup

Cook 1/2 cup raw millet in 1 1/3 cups water to yield 1 cup of cooked millet. When the water begins to boil, stir in the millet, cover and simmer 30 minutes.

Let the cooked millet cool. Then chop the nuts and fruits. The food processor may be used for this. Add the water and maple syrup (be sure to use pure maple syrup with no sugar added) and mix all these ingredients thoroughly with the millet. The food processor may be used for all the mixing if desired.

Form into balls, place on a plate, and refrigerate about two hours. They may be eaten like this or you may wish to dip them in a carob coating. If so, melt about 1/8 of a 1 pound block of natural beeswax. Add four tablespoons carob powder and four tablespoons honey. Stir until all ingredients are thoroughly mixed. Place a toothpick in each ball and dip the balls in the mixture. Leave the toothpick in, place back on the plate, and keep refrigerated until served.

Be flexible. Use your own choice of nuts and fruits. You may also substitute four tablespoons orange juice, four tablespoons apple juice, or two tablespoons of each for the water and maple syrup.

Challenge: Remember those old recipes you used to make -
the ones loaded with sugar, white flour, and saturated oils?
Use this page to rewrite them using wheat flour, olive oil or
butter, and honey. Substitute 2/3 to 3/4 cup honey for 1 cup
sugar. Do not alter the amount of oils and flour. For every
cup of flour, use 2 teaspoons baking soda and 1/4 teaspoon
salt.

Recipe _____

_____   _____
_____   _____
_____   _____
_____   _____

_____
_____
_____
_____
_____

Recipe _____

_____   _____
_____   _____
_____   _____
_____   _____

_____
_____
_____
_____
_____

.

Chapter 11

DELIGHTFUL

DRINKS

Whether therefore ye eat or drink, or whatsoever ye do, do all to the glory of God. I Corinthians 10:31.

Drinks

Water - Nothing takes the place of water. Your body consists of trillions of cells, 75% of these cells being water. Water activates the electrolytes in the body cells. It also plays an important role in enzyme activity. Water picks up wastes and toxins from the cells and carries them to the organs of elimination - the kidneys, bowels, lungs, and skin. Your body might expel up to one gallon of water every day through these organs. A small portion of it can be replaced by eating fresh fruits and vegetables, but I cannot stress enough the necessity of drinking water.

Get a good filtering system for your home if you don't already have one, and drink water! The average adult should drink six to eight glasses of water per day. Some need more, depending on the weather and physical activity.

Here's my recommendation for determining the minimum amount of water you should drink. Divide your body weight (in pounds) by 3. Drink at least that number of ounces per day. For instance, if you weigh 150 pounds, you should drink a minimum of 50 ounces of water per day in addition to any other drinks. In hot weather or if you exert yourself physically, you might need to divide your body weight by 2 and drink 75 ounces.

Listed on the following page are suggestions for other drinks in addition to water. I believe a person can be healthy if he eats properly and drinks plenty of water regardless of whether he drinks anything else. However, there are a number of healthful drinks which can be enjoyed during the day. Just don't try to substitute them for water. No other drink on earth can take the place of water.

Lemon Water - A glass of lemon water makes an excellent antioxidant. Combine the juice of one whole lemon with eight ounces of water. Sip it during the day or drink it with a meal. Tip: I do not think it wise to eat out very often, but when you do eat out, drink lemon water with your meal. This will help to expel toxins from your body. Let's face it - you don't really know what's in the food or how it was prepared.

Carrot Juice - Organic carrots have a pleasant, sweet taste. They are high in beta carotene, an excellent source of Vitamin A. The body stores beta carotene and converts it to Vitamin A as needed. Those who drink carrot juice do not blister easily when exposed to the sun. Vitamin A (carrots) and Vitamin D (sunshine) work well together.

Fruit Punch - Juice your own if possible. Combine apples, peaches, nectarines, pears, pineapple, strawberries, grapes - any combination you like. To make a "smoothie," blend a banana into your juice mixture.

Party Punch - If you need to make a large amount of punch for a party, buy bottles (not cans) of pure apple, grape, and pineapple juices with the pulp but containing no additives. Combine one quart apple juice, one quart grape juice, three cups filtered or distilled water, and one cup pineapple juice. Freeze two trays of the mixture to float in the remainder of the punch. It's pretty and tasty!

Milkshake - Place one cup of ice cream (pages 76-78,) two raw eggs, two teaspoons lecithin, and two cups rice milk in the blender. Add 1/4 cup nuts if desired. Blend well and drink immediately. This is enough to fill two large glasses. A small amount (about 1/4 teaspoon) of vanilla extract or another natural flavoring may be added if desired.

Chapter 12

SANDWICHES

Keep your sandwiches simple and eat them sparingly - especially meat sandwiches. They are much harder to digest than a balanced meal. Always eat a raw vegetable or a salad when you eat a sandwich. This will aid in digestion.

Sandwiches

Fast food sandwiches have become a vital part of the American diet, but they are far from healthful. A meal of green salad, beans, and rice is a much better choice. Overcome the fast food syndrome by preparing your meals so there will be sufficient leftovers for lunches. If you will do this on a consistent basis, your desire for fast food will totally diminish. I speak this from experience.

When my husband and I changed our diet because of his high blood pressure, our tastes soon changed. Within a few months, the fast food places we once frequented became repulsive to us. The smell was a stench in our nostrils.

Here are some suggestions for healthful sandwiches. Always eat a green salad or lettuce leaves with your sandwich. If you insist on a **sandwich spread**, blend together 1/2 cup cottage cheese and a celery stalk. Use on meat sandwiches.

Grilled cheese - Use whole grain bread, butter, and a brand of cheese without additives, preservatives, or dye.

Sloppy Joe - Make a sauce using the spaghetti sauce recipe on page 57. Add 1/2 cup of your favorite cooked beans with diced green peppers. Serve on whole grain bun or bread.

Meat sandwich - <u>Never</u> use "deli" meat or packaged meat from the grocery store cooler. Cook and freeze your own meat for sandwiches - turkey, chicken, and beef.

Scrambled egg sandwich - Soft scramble an egg in a little butter. Sprinkle with salt, pepper, and tarragon as desired.

Peanut butter / jelly - Use fresh peanut butter from a health food store and a 100% fruit spread with no refined sugar.

Chapter 13

WHAT'S ON

THE MENU?

amaranth   *almonds*   *beets*

pumpkin seeds   *raisins*   *carrots*   *lettuce*

tomato   *lentils*   *rice*

apple   **apricots**   **pineapple**   **banana**

bran muffins   **cucumber**   **celery**

7-Day Meal Plan

The following is a guideline for a 7-day meal plan which may be altered to meet your needs. Most families eat their main meal in the evening. However, if lunch is your family's largest meal, switch lunch and dinner.

If you work during the day, prepare lunch in advance and take it with you. Instead of using a microwave, try eating your food at room temperature. If your workplace is equipped to accomodate a small crockpot, invest in one for soup, beans, leftovers, etc. Plug it in about an hour before your lunch break, and your lunch will be deliciously warm!

Make an effort to eat a good breakfast. On a day that there is absolutely no time to make breakfast, eat a piece of fruit and a whole grain cereal.

Although it is not necessary to eat meat every day, I included it almost every day in the 7-day menu. Should you desire to eat meat only two or three times per week, substitute a legume and grain combination (see page 37) on the days you do not eat meat.

You will note that I suggest juice every morning for breakfast. If you do not have a juicer, I urge you to invest in one as soon as possible. Make your own juice from carrots, apples, oranges, grapefruit, pineapple, etc.

I purposely did not include dessert nor did I include sandwiches. Eat these foods sparingly. Keep in mind that the foods you need each day are fruits, vegetables, grains, legumes, nuts, and seeds.

Last but not least, remember to drink plenty of water every day.

Day 1

Breakfast: Applesauce - page 75
Oatmeal - page 16
2 tablespoons nuts and seeds - pages 9,11,16
8 oz. carrot juice

Lunch: Salad consisting of leaf lettuce, spinach,
            cabbage, broccoli, asparagus
Lentil soup - page 50

Dinner: 1 large lettuce leaf
Red beans and rice - page 40
Steamed broccoli, cauliflower, okra
Slice of whole grain bread or roll

Day 2

Breakfast: Grapefruit (or pineapple if available)
Grits with egg - page 18
2 tablespoons nuts and seeds
8 oz. apple juice

Lunch: Salad consisting of leaf lettuce, carrots,
            tomato, celery, cucumber
Barley-Bean soup - page 51

Dinner: An asparagus stalk
Spaghetti pie - page 60
Steamed vegetables (carrots, red skinned
            potatoes, green beans)
Bread with Mary's garlic spread - page 31

Day 3

Breakfast: A banana
2 tablespoons nuts and seeds
French toast served with pure maple syrup or
rice syrup - page 16
8 oz. carrot juice

Lunch: Salad consisting of leaf lettuce, spinach,
kale, carrots, celery
Baked sweet potato - page 47

Dinner:raw broccoli and cauliflower
brown rice and sweet peas - page 46
1 slice baked turkey - page 63
Bran muffin - page 27

Day 4

Breakfast: 1 cup melon (cantaloupe, watermelon, etc.)
2 tablespoons nuts and seeds
Bran muffin (left over from dinner)
8 oz. orange juice

Lunch: Salad consisting of leaf lettuce, spinach,
kale, celery, cauliflower, squash
Potato soup - page 52

Dinner:Several cucumber slices
Turkey/rice casserole or chicken/rice
casserole - pages 63,66
Navy beans - 38
Cornbread - page 28

Day 5

Breakfast: An orange
2 tablespoons nuts and seeds
Grits with egg - page 18
1 slice toast
8 oz. carrot juice

Lunch: Salad consisting of leaf lettuce, tomatoes,
cabbage, celery, cucumber
Cream of carrot soup - page 52

Dinner:1 large lettuce leaf
Lentil/rice casserole - page 39
Baked squash - 46
Millet bread - page 28

Day 6

Breakfast: An apple
2 tablespoons nuts and seeds
Oatmeal - 16
1 slice toast
8 oz. grapefruit juice

Lunch: Salad consisting of leaf lettuce, spinach,
kale, celery, cucumber
Vegetable stew - 44

Dinner:Sliced tomato
Broiled fish - 69
Brown rice (page 40) seasoned with
oregano, basil, and liquid aminos
Steamed broccoli - 43
Bread with Mary's garlic spread - page 31

Day 7

Breakfast: 1 cup melon
                    2 tablespoons nuts and seeds
                    1 slice toast
                    8 oz. carrot juice

Lunch: Salad consisting of leaf lettuce, squash,
                            carrots, broccoli, cauliflower
                    Split pea soup - page 50

Dinner: Sliced cucumber
                    Turkey patties - page 63
                    Lentils - page 39
                    Quinoa - page 38
                    Slice of whole grain bread or roll

If you are accustomed to snacking, try to limit your snacks to mid morning and mid afternoon. Bedtime snacks hinder proper assimilation of foods eaten during the day.

Eat one or two servings per day of fruit. Fruit juice is considered a serving of fruit.

Eat five to seven servings of vegetables per day. If you make a large salad consisting of a variety of vegetables, this may compensate for as many as five vegetable servings.

Include approximately 2 tablespoons of raw, unprocessed nuts and seeds in your every day diet.

Eat one or two generous servings of legumes and two to three servings of grains every day.

As you incorporate more healthful foods into your diet, you will find that you have no desire, no time, and no room for harmful processed foods. Try it!

Now that you have made meals with Mary, make a list of your favorite foods and incorporate them into your every day plan for healthful eating. Remember, your every day diet should include fruits, vegetables, nuts, seeds, legumes, and grains.

Vegetables (7 servings per day)   **Fruits (1 to 2 servings per day)**

_____   _____

_____   _____

_____   _____

_____   _____

_____   _____

_____   _____

_____

Nuts (1 tablespoon per day)   **Seeds (1 tablespoon per day)**

_____   _____

_____   _____

_____   _____

_____   _____

Legumes (1 to 2 servings)   **Whole Grains (2 to 3 servings)**

_____   _____

_____   _____

_____   _____

_____   _____

_____   _____

_____

Chapter 14

IT'S YOUR
CHOICE

*.....Choose you this day whom ye will serve.....but as for me and my
house, we will serve the Lord. Joshua 24:15*

It's Your Choice

I can think of only one thing more important than your health - that is your salvation. Your health is a major determining factor in how well you enjoy life on this earth; what you do with Jesus Christ determines where you will spend eternity.

Jesus Christ is God's Son. According to John 3:16, God loved you and me so much that He gave His only begotten Son to shed His precious blood and die on a cruel cross so we might have eternal life. In order to claim this eternal life, we must recognize the fact that we are depraved sinners and doomed for eternity in the lake of fire forever if we reject God's Son as our Saviour. Romans 3:23 teaches that *all have sinned and come short of the glory of God.* Romans 6:23 clearly states that *the wages of sin is death but the gift of God is eternal life through Jesus Christ our Lord.*

Now let's read Romans 10:9,10. *That is thou shalt confess with thy mouth the Lord Jesus, and shalt believe in thine heart that God hath raised him from the dead thou shalt be saved. For with the heart man believeth unto righteousness and with the mouth confession is made unto salvation.*

Just as you must decide for yourself to eat healthful meals, you must decide for yourself what you will do with Jesus. If you wish to accept Him as your own personal Savior, won't you take the time right now to pray a simple prayer acknowledging your sinful, depraved condition, thank Him for His death on the cross, and ask Him to forgive your sins, come into your heart, and save you?

All sin was paid for on the cross. There is no need for you to carry your burden of sin any longer. Give it to Jesus who is crucified, risen, and coming again.

If you have accepted Jesus as your own personal Savior as a result of reading this, or if you are already a Christian, I urge you to read your Bible every day. Mark passages, study them, and pray for understanding. This will enable you to grow spiritually. It will also make you aware that your body is now the Lord's body (I Corinthians 6:19,20).

You will find that the Bible has much to say about food and how to care for the body. Daniel 1:8 is one example. Young Daniel purposed in his heart that he would not defile himself with the portion of the king's meat nor the wine which he drank. Three other young men, Shadrach, Meshach, and Abednego, joined Daniel in this decision. Daniel requested of his superiors that he and his friends be given pulse to eat and water to drink. This "pulse" was food that grew out the ground - legumes, grains, vegetables, fruits, nuts, and seeds.

The pulse that they ate was rich in phytochemicals, enzymes, and antioxidants. Grown in the soil and harvested when ripe, it contained a perfect balance of these precious nutrients. God in His wisdom designed our bodies to get vitamins and minerals from foods - not pills. It was no mere coincidence that at the end of ten days Daniel and his friends were healthier than all the children who ate the king's meat.

I find no indication that this passage is forbidding meat consumption; yet, it is made clear that the fruits and vegetables the Hebrew children ate had far more nutritional value than the king's meat. Exactly what did the king's meat consist of? Let's relate that incident to the American diet.

These were young men, probably teenagers. What do our teens, our children, our adults, eat today in this land of plenty? Since our nation has become industrialized, we have strayed from preparing our own meals. Unfortunately, the American way is to find a fast food restaurant or thaw a frozen dinner and proceed to the many demands crowding our lives. Are these demands more important than our health? If so, let's forget the natural foods and continue eating the processed foods that will poison our bodies and cause disease.

I fully believe that the popular American diet is a tool of the devil to make Christians sick. What you put into your body becomes a part of you. It is impossible to function properly when your body is filled with indigestible chemicals.

It is sad but true that many Christians try to convince themselves that God will sanctify whatever they eat according to I Timothy 4:4,5 *For every creature of God is good, and nothing to be refused, if it be received with thanksgiving: For it is sanctified by the word of God and prayer.*

Read the whole context of these verses. Verse 4 specifies every creature of God, referring to animals, fish, and birds, not hot dogs and bologna which are leftover scraps fit for only the garbage can. Don't deceive yourself. These verses offer no more assurance of sanctifying foods that contain harmful chemicals than Philippians 4:19 gives you permission to intentionally miss work and expect God to supply all your needs according to His riches in glory.

I am not suggesting that we offend others by refusing certain foods. Use discretion. Let others know that you make every effort to eat healthful meals. This can be done graciously.

It isn't popular to refuse a piece of cake at a birthday party or a wedding reception. *Just one slice won't hurt anything, will it?* One slice? How frequently? Would it make a difference if you could see refined sugar leeching nutrients from your body in order to digest itself?

Are you afraid your children will be "different" and not have friends if you tell them hot dogs, sandwich meats, sugar, and soft drinks are bad for them? Haven't you taught them not to cross the street without watching for oncoming vehicles and not to play with rattlesnakes? Why not be concerned about their health? Teach them self discipline at an early age. *He that hath no rule over his own spirit is like a city broken down and without walls.* Proverbs 25:28.

When there is a social function, contribute a healthful dish. Make an effort to establish good eating habits in your area. Encourage family and friends to join you. Don't be discouraged when others show skepticism or rebellion. Be patient. Perseverance pays. Let your family know that you love them and that you care about their health. III John 2 puts health on a very high level. If God cares that much about our health, shouldn't we take it seriously?

If you have made a decision to accept Christ as your own personal Savior as a result of reading this chapter, I would like to hear from you. I would also like to know if the information in this book has enlightened and encouraged you to change your eating habits and enjoy good health.

If you have resolved to make an honest effort to eat a healthful diet, please let me know so I can pray for you daily. I ask two things of you. First, do not cheat as you will only be cheating yourself. Second, stay with the program a full six months. You will be glad you did. God bless you!

For more information about nutrition, contact
Mary Hughen
The Nutrition Mission
1825 Morgan Cemetery Road
Molino, Florida 32577
850-587-5680

Glossary of Ingredients and Terms

Amaranth - A whole grain which contains an excellent balance of the amino acids. Unlike most grains, it is high in both lysine and methionine.

Arrowroot - An somewhat starchy herb used to thicken soups, stews, gravies.

Baking powder - Enhances rising of bread. Use a brand which does not contain aluminum. Aluminum in the diet has been linked with colitis, stomach ulcers, and asthma. The brand I use is Rumford.

Barley - A whole grain mentioned favorably in the Bible. Highly regarded as having important medicinal properties.

Basil - An herb used to flavor pasta dishes, vegetables, and soups. Has medicinal properties.

Carob - Fruit from a small evergreen tree. The fruit grows into a flat, dark brown leathery pod (legume) about one foot long. The beans are roasted and ground into a fine powder similar to cocoa. Carob contains calcium and phosphorus.

Celery - Chop or dice for use in salads. Chop or blend for use in soups, casseroles, etc. Contains natural salt.

Chives - An herb which adds flavor to potato soup and carrot soup as well as other dishes.

Cinnamon - A spice used for flavoring apples, sweet potatoes, and breads.

Flour - Always use a whole grain flour.

Garlic - High in iodine and sulfur. Health professionals recommend it as an aid for regulating blood pressure. Adds flavor to pasta dishes, vegetables, and soups.

Ginger - Has been known to relieve upset stomach and indigestion. Add 1/4 to 1/2 teaspoon to meat dishes to help digest the meat.

Gluten - Basically wheat flour with the starch removed. Gluten enhances the rising of breads.

Lecithin granules - Use in fruit salad, cereal, cakes, and ice cream. It has its own distinctive flavor - somewhat like fruit. Lecithin enables fats, such as cholesterol, to be dispersed in water and removed from the body. Available in health food stores.

Leeks - A favorite vegetable for soups and broths because of their delicate onion flavor.

Liquid Aminos - A sauce made from pure soybeans. Contains 16 amino acids. Sodium is naturally occurring. Tastes somewhat like soy sauce. Adds flavor to salads, soups, casseroles, meat dishes, and vegetables. Available in health food stores.

Millet - A whole grain, favorably mentioned in the Bible.

Olive Oil - Buy pure, cold-pressed (unheated) extra virgin olive oil.

Onion - Rich in Vitamin C. One of the earliest known food medicines used for colds and catarrhal disorders. Eat raw or cooked with meat, vegetables, pasta, and other dishes.

Oregano - An herb used to flavor pasta dishes, vegetables, chicken, grains, legumes, and soups. A digestive aid.

Parsley - An herb rich in chlorophyll content. Adds flavor and decor to grains and casseroles.

Quinoa - A whole grain about the size of a mustard seed, high in protein. When well done, grains will be translucent, and the outer germ ring will separate.

Sage - A well known seasoning for chicken, turkey, all poultry dishes, soups, etc. A strong sage tea has been used successfully as an excellent gargle for tonsillitis or ulcers in the mouth or throat.

Spelt - A dark wheat, referred to in the Bible as "fitches."

Stevia - A natural sweetener 30 to 100 times sweeter than sugar. High in chromium which helps to establish a good balance of blood sugar. A small amount goes a long way. All diabetics should use this.

Tarragon - An herb which adds flavor to scrambled egg sandwiches, meat patties, and grains.

Thyme - An herb used to flavor pasta dishes, vegetables, salads, and soups. May have a calming effect on the nerves.

Xanthan Gum - Produced by fermentation and ground to a fine powder. Use sparingly as a thickener for ice cream, pastries, soups, etc.

REFERENCES

The Holy Bible, Authorized King James Version.

Diane Campbell, *Step By Step To Natural Food,* Clearwater, Fl: CC Publishers, 1979.

Dr. Edward Howell, *Enzyme Nutrition,* Wayne, NJ: Avery Publishing Group, Inc., 1985.

Andrew Weil, M.D., *Natural, Health, Natural Medicine,* Boston, NY: Houghton Mifflin Co., 1995.

Harvey and Marilyn Diamond, *Fit For Life, II,* New York NY: Warner Books, 1987.

Jethro Kloss, *Back To Eden,* 12th edition. Loma Linda, Ca: Back To Eden Publishing Co., 1995.

Louise Tenney, M.H., *Today's Herbal Health,* 3rd edition. Provo, Ut: Woodland Books, 1992.

Fred C. Hess, *Chemistry Made Simple,* Revised by Arthur L. Thomas, Ph.D., New York, NY: Doubleday, 1984.

Rudolph Ballentine, M.D., *Diet & Nutrition,* Honesdale, Pa: The Himalayan International Institute, 1984.

INDEX

Scarlett ~~Monro~~ Monroe